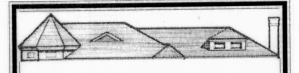

Southold Free Library

In Honor Of

Dr. Glenn Geelhoed

M2H Board of Directors
January 2014

Advance Praise for *Mission to Heal*

"I had no idea that teaching surgical techniques, or as Dr. Geelhoed calls it, the 'indigeniza-tion' of a skill to the world's 'bottom billion' could in itself make quality surgical care go viral! Read this book, share it with your colleagues, join the Glenn Geelhoed Mission to Heal fan club and give hope to those who previously had none."
—Jerry M. Kekos, CEO, National Institute of First Assisting (NIFA)®

"*Mission to Heal* is an amazing account of selfless dedication, the utmost definition of philan-thropy and volunteerism. Mission seekers and volunteers can take lessons from the book's chapters, which contain templates and examples of countless scenarios one would face under such circumstances. Glenn demonstrates good judgment and humility in upholding the Hippocratic oath and seeking help from other physicians in order to best serve the patient."
—Oheneba Boachie-Adjei, MD, Professor of Orthopaedic Surgery, Weill Medical College of Cornell University; Attending Orthopaedic Surgeon & Chief, Scoliosis Service, Hospital for Special Surgery; Past President, Scoliosis Research Society (2008-2009); Founder & President, FOCOS (www.orthofocos.org)

"Dr. Glenn Geelhoed has chosen to leave American soil to provide medical care to some of the most impoverished people on the planet. And motivate and teach hundreds of students on the way. Read this for inspiration."
—Rick Hodes, MD, MACP, medical director of Ethiopia for the American Jewish Joint Distribution Committee

"Dr. Glenn Geelhoed has the heart for the medical and surgical needs of the poor of the world. In the eighteen years that we have worked together in the Philippines, he has brought with him many physicians and medical students from the United States who Dr. Geelhoed hopes will carry on his passion to heal the poor. He believes, as I do, that teaching, training and supporting indigenous doctors, nurses and paramedical personnel is the key to providing medical care to the people of that country. I wholeheartedly endorse Dr. Glenn Geelhoed's book, *Mission to Heal*."
—Alfredo V. Casino, MD, FACS, president, American Foundation To Aid The Poor

"Give a man a fish and you feed him for a day. Teach a man to fish and you feed him for a lifetime. Dr. Geelhoed's story shows that teaching is as important as healing in delivering healthcare to indigenous communities around the world."

—MICHAEL MARQUARDT, director of the Executive Leadership Doctoral Program at George Washington University; president of the World Institute of Action Learning

"*Mission to Heal* and Glenn Geelhoed's personal sense of mission and vision to serve is the story of a remarkable man accomplishing for the 'bottom billion' what few ever dare to attempt. The reader will be astonished and bewildered by the passion and laser focus of Glenn's life and work; those in search of helpful coordinates for their own life's work will find here an emblematic and inspiring account to spur them onward."

—THE REV. DR. PETER J. KELLEY, pastor, First Presbyterian Church of Southold, New York

"*Mission to Heal* is one part medical textbook, one part political and geographic primer, and every other part adventurer's travel log. In life and in text, Dr. Geelhoed's retelling is comprehensive, multifaceted, and never boring."

—THE REV. MARGARET J. JENISTA, Washington DC Christian Reformed Church

Mission *to* Heal

*Sharing Medical Knowledge
at Africa's Pole of Inaccessibility*

DR. GLENN W. GEELHOED

GREENLEAF
BOOK GROUP PRESS

Published by Greenleaf Book Group Press
Austin, Texas
www.gbgpress.com

Distributed by Greenleaf Book Group LLC

For ordering information or special discounts for bulk purchases, please contact
Greenleaf Book Group LLC at PO Box 91869, Austin, TX 78709, 512.891.6100.

Design and composition by Greenleaf Book Group LLC
Cover design by Greenleaf Book Group LLC
Cover image © iStockphoto/austinmann

Publisher's Cataloging-In-Publication Data
Geelhoed, Glenn W., 1942-
  Mission to heal : sharing medical knowledge at Africa's pole of inaccessibility/Glenn W.
Geelhoed. —1st ed.
   p. : ill. ; cm.
  Issued also as an ebook.
  ISBN: 978-1-62634-028-2
  1. Missions, Medical—Central African Republic. 2. Indigenous peoples—Medical
care—Central African Republic. 3. Medical care—Central African Republic. I. Title.

R722 .G44 2014
362.1/096741   2013949639

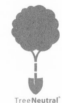

Part of the Tree Neutral® program, which offsets the number of trees
consumed in the production and printing of this book by taking proactive
steps, such as planting trees in direct proportion to the number of trees
used: www.treeneutral.com

TreeNeutral®

Printed in the United States of America on acid-free paper

13 14 15 16 17 18   10 9 8 7 6 5 4 3 2 1

First Edition

For my fellow students who seek to learn, even those who may never have been in school, and the transformation that we celebrate on each side of this relationship in our shared Mission to Heal.

Contents

Foreword

In purchasing this book, you have bought a ticket for a unique and compelling journey with Dr. Glenn Geelhoed and Mission To Heal (M2H), a 501(c)(3) nonprofit organization created to support medical missions to remote corners of the world—places most people never have the chance to experience, where most Westerners never go, and where there exists a great need for medical surgical care.

On your journey, you'll experience firsthand a world painted vividly by Dr. Geelhoed—parts of Africa where war and famine persist and where only the bravest venture. Humanitarianism is not dead; there are those who give back and back and back. M2H and Dr. Geelhoed have been going on medical surgical missions for over forty years now, giving much-needed medical care to those who would not otherwise receive it, the often forgotten people of the world.

None of the volunteers in M2H or those who go on these medical surgical missions receive anything in the way of monetary remuneration; their reward is the feeling of helping another human being in need. Indeed 100 percent of the proceeds from the sale of this book go toward funding future medical surgical missions.

Mission To Heal has impacted thousands of people in ways both tangible and intangible. Some feel more connected with life and get a degree of personal satisfaction from assisting in advancing the work of Dr. Geelhoed and M2H. Others, particularly mission team participants, enjoy transformational learning experiences and gain lessons in resilience, resourcefulness, and the ability to find joy and purpose even under dire circumstances. Of course, those most impacted are the patients, those men, women, and children who received medical treatment and either had their lives saved or their quality of life enhanced beyond their own imaginations.

M2H exists only because of the generosity of so many who give to M2H with their donations of time and money. Visit M2H at www.Mission2Heal. org to learn more about this unique organization and how you can become a part of it and future missions.

Now sit back, turn on the light, and get ready for the journey of a lifetime! Enjoy the ride with renowned surgeon Dr. Glenn Geelhoed and the team of M2H volunteers! You will not be unchanged.

—John McLaurin,
   Chairman, M2H Board of Directors

Prologue

Our fourth operating day in the Central African Republic (CAR) January visit was much like the others. When we had landed in Obo at dawn the day before, after an exhausting two days in Zemio, seventy miles to the west, we were presented with a mind-numbing list of 320 patients—and we had just two days to see them all, operating on many of them. And so now, on our last full operating day in the country, we faced a crowd of potential patients, gathered in family groups outside the mud-brick clinic.

A portion of the thatch ceiling of the small room we used for consultations had collapsed, and Jon Hildebrandt, our pilot, was working with a local man to repair it. Jon had found somebody who spoke Kiswahili, a rarity in the southeast corner of the CAR. Most of the indigenous population are of the Zande tribe and so speak Pazande. Fortunately, we could continue to work in the room while Jon worked above us; it was the dry season in equatorial January, and no rain threatened our examinations.

Ambroise Soungouza, director of the Zemio clinic, had traveled to Obo with me, and he called the next patient in. The figure of a woman of healthy adult size, her hair braided in rows, stepped through the doorway. She seemed young to me, but her age was hard to judge—her left hand held up a scarf to cover the lower portion of her face. I'm not certain I noticed at the time, but later I realized that the scarf had been covered with flies. In the dry season, that could mean only one thing: It was damp.

Ambroise greeted her in Pazande, and she turned and directed a steady, intense gaze at me. Often the women I see in these remote parts of the world are shy with me and won't make or maintain eye contact, but not this woman. As she took a few steps forward in the limited space we had, she held my gaze. She seemed to be assessing me, although it should have been the other way around. In the next moment, I understood why.

Her left hand moved and the scarf fell away from her face. Where her lower lip should have been was a massive irregular growth that had turned her lip into the petals of a grotesque flower, obscuring her entire lower jaw. The surface of it was covered with bumps and sores. Saliva ran over the growth; there was no barrier to keep it in her mouth and it was clear that the tumor had created a salivary fistula, or an abnormal opening between the salivary glands and the place where the skin of the lower lip and chin should have held the saliva in. I had never seen anything quite like this disfiguring disease.

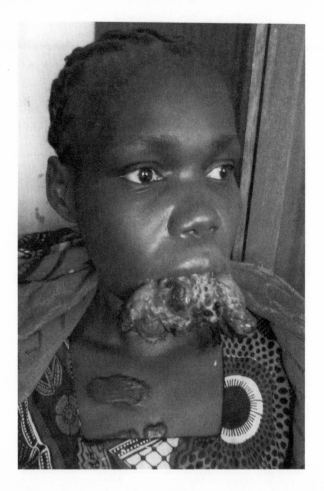

Rather than casting her eyes away from mine in embarrassment, she remained focused on me, watching my reaction closely. Would I respond like others had, with shock, revulsion, even fear? My response certainly wasn't what she had anticipated. Her eyes widened as I grabbed my camera, stepped forward, and snapped her photo—my rudimentary form of imaging and patient record keeping. I then immediately called one of my students, Dan Vryhof, in from the adjoining room—our "operating theater." Dan paused when he turned the corner, speechless for half a moment, but quickly recovered and became the model clinician.

Ambroise explained that the woman's name was Flore and began to translate my questions as I examined her. The growth was so exposed that I spent only a moment on it before jumping straight to her neck and chest. Were her lymph nodes involved, and had this growth spread, or metastasized, to other parts of her body, particularly the lungs? I described my exam to Dan and Ambroise as I went, explaining what my fingers were searching for in her neck, what I was listening for as she breathed.

Ambroise gathered her history, with comments from Flore and her brother and sister, who had accompanied her to the clinic. We learned that she was thirty-five years old, a widow (her husband had died of a wasting disease a few months earlier), and the mother of five young children. *Five children who might soon become orphans*, I thought.

Yet I found nothing in Flore's neck or chest.

I listened to the details coming from Ambroise, interjecting questions here and there. I was perplexed by what I was finding, so I asked, "How long has this tumor been present?"

Ambroise translated, Flore responded, and Ambroise gave me the answer. Four weeks.

That can't be possible, I thought. I asked Ambroise to ask the family. Flore's brother and sister responded that it was closer to three weeks.

That growth rate was a bad indicator. Flore was suffering from a malignant growth, a carcinoma that could be clinically staged as a T3N0M0 tumor—T3 meaning that the tumor was larger than 5 centimeters, N0 meaning that the nodes were not clinically involved (no painless swelling or unusual induration was palpable), and M0 meaning that there was no sign of distant metastasis. Yet she was young and otherwise seemed healthy. Given the pace of growth, it was astounding that the cancer had not spread. Still, if we did nothing, her five dependents would quickly become orphans, possibly within a week.

I began to realize that we might have a tiny window of opportunity. If the tumor could be resected, we might be able to deliver a miracle. "We have to try to save her," I said to the skeptical team.

In many parts of the world, those words would have spurred the rapid activity of entire teams—a surgical team, an oncological team, social workers to ensure the welfare of the children involved, hospital administrators, and so on. But we were not in one of those places. We were near the African pole of inaccessibility, a geographer's term for the most remote point in a region or on a continent, the farthest from any sea, navigable river, or other mode of access. In Africa, that point is at 5.65°N 26.17°E, near Obo, in the Central African Republic.

Standing in Obo, you might find it difficult to think of the area as the most remote in Africa. In fact, it sometimes seems more like a market for cultural exchange. While the region is inhabited predominantly by the Zande people, one of the primary tribes of central Africa, for years other tribal peoples have intermittently spilled over the porous borders around this pole of inaccessibility. Surges of refugees have moved in and out of the CAR from the newly minted Republic of South Sudan and from Uganda. The Fulani, Islamic nomadic herders from the west African Sahel, have been moving into the area in search of grazing lands as the Sahara Desert creeps down the continent. The area is supposed to be a preserve to support the hunter-gatherer and small-scale farming lifestyle of the Azande (the plural of Zande, used to refer to the people as a group), but like many of the nations in central Africa, the CAR is a failed nation-state with little control over its borders. And this increases the impression of inaccessibility.

That inaccessibility was precisely why I was in the CAR. I have been conducting medical missions in Africa, and on almost every other continent, since 1968, and for decades have returned to treat the Zande people in Assa, a village about sixty-eight miles southwest of Obo that was in Zaire until the name of that putative nation-state changed to the Democratic Republic of the Congo (DRC). (Assa is not to be confused with Asa, DRC, much farther to the south.) In the late 1980s, this remote region was overrun by the spillover of the Hutu-Tutsi conflict in Rwanda far to the east. Later it was again disturbed by the civil war of the Congolese, with Laurent Kabila attempting an overthrow of Mobutu Sese Seko, the entrenched "president for life."

But in 2009, the people of Assa again fled their homes, escaping the marauding Lord's Resistance Army (LRA) that had grown out of strife between northern and southern Uganda. The LRA emerged from a faction of the Ugandan army but had become more of a pseudoreligious cult, with a stated goal of establishing a theocratic state based on the Ten Commandments and the traditions of the Acholi people of northern Uganda and South Sudan. But the actions of its leader, Joseph Kony, and of its members belie that beatific intent. Kony seems focused on escaping capture and surviving on the backs of indigenous people in Uganda, the Democratic Republic of the Congo, and now the CAR and the Republic of South Sudan. Because the LRA has been responsible for the displacement of more than two million people, the conscription of more than sixty thousand child soldiers, and terrible war crimes, including murder, mutilation, and rape, Kony is now a hunted man.

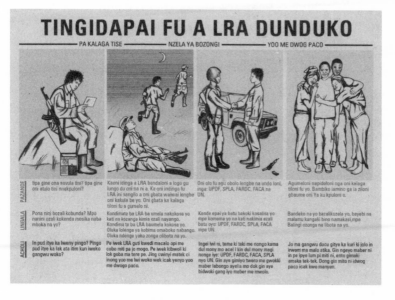

I found this leaflet in the forest around Zemio. The African Union dropped these in the area to encourage LRA members to give themselves up, promising that they would be reunited with their families.

As bands of the LRA spread across the northern DRC, murdering and abducting people from small, remote villages, the families of Assa fled into the surrounding rainforest. Organized by my longtime Zande friend Jean Marco, they crossed the Mbomou River into the CAR, officially becoming refugees when they crossed an international border; had they stayed and tried to subsist in the bush near their plundered DRC villages, they would have been classified as internally displaced persons (IDPs). Amazingly, within a few short years, they built a new village in the town of Zemio. Nobody had stopped them at the border or prevented them from developing the village.

I came to the CAR first and foremost because I was anxious to see my friends from Assa, the people for whom I had been caring for twenty years. Theirs was not the only refugee camp in the region, but they had established it without sanction and with little help. They are one of the most resourceful groups I have ever met.

A nation with porous borders like the CAR's is an ideal refuge for people who are forced to flee their homelands—and for the armies who forced them to flee. The LRA is active in the CAR, performing acts of violence just to show they can; the Assa refugees still live in fear. But the LRA are being hunted, so they avoid larger towns like Zemio and Obo, relying on what they can plunder and the people they can abduct from the smaller villages. And a joint action of the African Union, led by the Uganda People's Defence Force (UPDF) troops and the US Africa Command (AFRICOM) for support, is in force in the eastern CAR to try to root out the LRA. They at least have been successful in surveillance, which is curbing some of the violence and abductions.

Thus, the CAR has three foreign forces—the LRA, the UPDF, and AFRICOM—acting within its borders, with little influence or control from the country's faraway central government, which has more than enough troubles of its own near the capital, Bangui. This is the second reason I led a team to the CAR—we go where there is the greatest need. And in this country where the so-called host government provides no security for its own people and where there is no infrastructure for medical services, particularly for refugees, need is great.

It had taken almost three years of planning to get our team of students and surgical assistants to this point, which is surprising only because I have been traveling all around this region for decades. We had wasted valuable, scarce resources and time in one failed attempt to get into the CAR the year before. I still clench my jaw in frustration when I remember spending a week in January 2011 paying for a chartered airplane, its belly full of surgical supplies, to sit on the gravel and grit of a UPDF airfield named Nzara in South Sudan near the border with the CAR. Due to an administrative quagmire caused by the chaos after CAR elections, we waited in vain for clearance to fly into the country.

But we had made it eventually, a year later, and because we did, Flore might have a chance to be saved.

When I said those fateful words—"We have to try to save her"—Ambroise immediately responded, "That isn't possible." Flore required a major operation, and Ambroise saw that it wasn't something we could accomplish with the limited supplies in our makeshift operating room. There were too many hurdles to count, but at the top of the list was the fact that we didn't have the ability to deliver general anesthesia or to intubate with an endotracheal tube, both of which would be necessary. We were operating on the fringes of surgical safety, pushing the envelope by doing major operations—including thyroidectomies, hysterectomies, and hernia repairs—with local and spinal anesthetics. We needed to get Flore to a surgical center, which meant flying her out.

"Jon," I called up through the hole in the ceiling, "is there room for one more in the plane?" We were already half-packed with one foot out the door and were planning to fly out early the next morning in the Cessna 208 Caravan, which seated ten but also had to carry bags and possibly barrels of fuel.

"It wouldn't be just one more," he replied, and I realized what he meant. Flore would be in the hospital for weeks and then would need to travel back to her family. She would need an escort and somebody to translate and provide care.

We began rapid discussions. If we could get her out, where would we take her? Where did they have the capability to do an operation of this magnitude? Certainly not in the CAR, where there are very few doctors and almost no specialists, even in the capital of Bangui. Our next stop was Kenya, where I would be catching a flight to the Philippines. Kijabe Hospital in Kenya had rotating specialists from the United States, and it was a part of the Africa Inland Mission (AIM) network. Much of my work in Africa was in the ersatz clinics of the AIM mission stations (usually set up for midwifery only) and we were traveling via AIM AIR, the organization's charter flight service. I knew the fact that I had an account with AIM would help ensure that Flore got the care she needed at Kijabe, despite the fact that she obviously could not pay for it.

But first we had to find out if they would take her, if they had the ability to treat her, if there was a surgeon in residence who could perform the operation. Curiously, there is a cell phone tower in Obo, recently erected as part of the US Special Operations Forces (SOF) encampment. Obo and the surrounding area might be geographically inaccessible, but at this moment, magically, it was not technologically inaccessible.

Jon handed me his cell phone. "It has four minutes on the SIM card," he said.

It's not easy to carry a woman—a passportless citizen—who has never left the pole of inaccessibility, or been on an airplane or likely any vehicle more complex than a bicycle, across the borders of three nations to get her access to specialized medical care. And I had four minutes to work it out.

I called Kijabe Hospital and said that I wished to report a patient in urgent need of an operation. I had heard that Dr. Peter Bird, an Australian surgeon, had been in residence at Kijabe, and so I asked if he or his deputy might speak with me about a critical referral from outside of Kijabe and Kenya. It took them a minute and a half to get Dr. Bird on the phone. I quickly began explaining the situation, and from a few of his comments, I could tell Dr. Bird might have thought I was a wealthy tourist who had taken pity on a hard case I'd seen on the side of the road as I whisked through on a guided expedition. But my profession became clear as I began running the details, as a surgeon would: "I have a thirty-five-year-old female with a T3N0M0 squamous cell carcinoma at the mucocutaneous junction, and a resulting salivary fistula, in need of an extensive resection." The extent of our negotiations before the phone died was that he agreed to see her. Apparently, before he realized I wasn't on the line anymore, he explained that he would see her as long as I agreed to be responsible for all costs related to her treatment.

Ambroise and Flore's family were scrambling to work out the rest of the details. Who would accompany her? Who would take care of her children? Blaise, her brother, would go as her chaperone and translator, and Ambroise would go as her caregiver. Her sister agreed to care for Flore's children, despite the fact that she had her own and would be caring for Flore's for who knew how long. The youngest was still nursing and would have to be weaned overnight.

Flore had no identifying paperwork of any kind and we had only eight hours before we were supposed to be wheels-up. Fortunately, there was a prefecture commissioner in Obo who could provide letters stating who Flore was, why she was traveling—although she carried proof enough on her face—and that she would be returning to the CAR. The intent to return was a crucial element of the paperwork. There would be no enthusiasm at the Kenyan airport for a needy CAR citizen who hoped to take advantage of whatever scarce human health and welfare resources the country might furnish. The immigration of an undocumented Zande woman, accompanied by two Zande men, one not even related to her, would not happen unless we guaranteed her repatriation following her medical treatment.

Somehow, Flore's supporters pulled the details together, and early the next day, we all loaded into the Cessna 208. I strapped her into the seat behind mine, the copilot's "right seat." As we took off, her eyes widened above the scarf that still covered her mouth, and I reached back to hold her hand. She gripped it tightly and stared out the window, barely blinking as she took in the vast world beneath us on the twenty-minute flight from Obo to Zemio. Her brother, Blaise, also stared at the rainforest below as he sailed off into the unknown, recognizing only that this was his sister's one slim hope and trusting in the help of strangers, at a scale they could hardly comprehend.

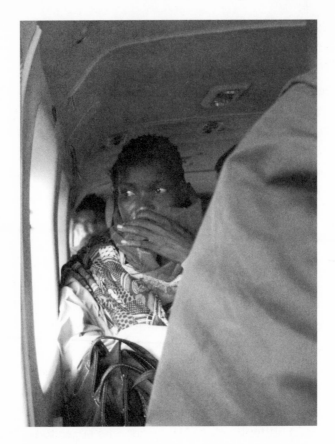

Despite Flore's desperation, her mad scramble to prepare to leave, her life-threatening illness, her lack of certainty as to what was to come, and her lack of control over her medical or economic or diplomatic circumstances, she had chosen to put her best foot forward, to go out trying. During the night, she had painted her toenails in preparation for her entry onto the global stage.

What we did for Flore was unprecedented. Our medical missions, now operating as a nonprofit organization called Mission to Heal (or M2H), are fraught with difficult decisions regarding all the patients we can or cannot help. Rarely, very rarely, we find a patient who we feel should be transported out of his or her world to a more developed medical center for treatment, a patient who has a treatable condition (a tumor that could be resected, for instance) with a high likelihood of survival. Every bit of life in these places is a judgment call; the nuances are not trivial. With Flore, they included the fact that she was the single parent of five children. But it's possible to arrive with a budget of $10,000, spend four times that amount on the first patient, and not improve his or her life at all, or anybody else's for that matter. We see hundreds of patients, and often our response is "You can live with this" or "You will certainly die from this." Comfort care is what we, and they, accept. Whom to treat when not all can be treated is a major ethical dilemma. The resources for the many can be easily diverted to investment in a few, even though some of those patients might have very long shots at a rehabilitated life. Is not this the same moral dilemma in the collision of the first world's redundancy against the third world's insatiable needs, a dilemma recurring daily whether within or outside national boundaries?

Some might ask why we have the right to make such decisions. There is only one reason: There is nobody else here to make them.

Although many people believe that these local populations are inaccessible, that they cannot be helped—and I have been told just that numerous times—I have reached them time and again, and I hope that I have helped. In fact, we made two trips to Zemio and Obo in 2012, the first in January, when we met Flore, and the second in June. And we plan to return again soon. But not to act as angels of mercy, swooping in to rescue the sick. While we certainly treat the local populations during our missions, it has never been my goal to become their primary caregiver. Of course, that would be unsustainable—how many continents can I be on at once, or even in a single year, particularly given the expense of transporting a team and supplies to some of the most remote locations on earth? More important, this endeavor would not help these people in the long term.

The primary goal of my work has always been to train indigenous caregivers, like Ambroise, by empowering and supplying them with skills and equipment to carry on a sustainable, local health-care program. In some locations, it has worked better than others. I'm sharing the story of my missions to the CAR because the local clinics are thriving there, thanks to the continued hard work of the indigenous health-care workers. My responsibility to them is to try to teach them good judgment. If I do something foolish, the danger is that it will become enshrined as normal care. Taking Flore to Kenya was a very risky choice. If treating her turned out to be foolhardy, the observers would think they should do everything remotely possible for everybody, no matter the cost or consequences.

Instead, I work to continually learn an important lesson from the local workers and to teach this lesson to the students who travel with me. These people have adapted to considerable resource constraints, and they have found ways to do a whole lot more with very much less. That is a skill we need to learn and teach.

I hope we will continue to teach and learn at clinics in the CAR. But as of this writing, it is difficult to know their future, or when we will be able to return, despite the plans we already have in development. In addition to the turmoil I've described, the CAR is in the midst of a military coup, the most recent in a long string of such governmental "transitions." Séléka, a rebel coalition led by Michel Djotodia, has taken over the capital of Bangui, ousting President François Bozizé, who has fled the country. From a Western perspective, this may seem like a dramatic turn of events, and we are certainly concerned for our friends in Zemio and Obo. But the Bozizé government had so little influence on or control over the eastern part of the country that the coup may have little effect on the lives of the people who live there—if the violence is limited.

For the refugees from Assa, the situation is even more tenuous. While the CAR experiences political upheaval, the DRC, their home country, faces the same situation. Since a troubled election in 2010, a rebel group called M23 has become active, particularly in the eastern DRC, near the country's border with Uganda and Rwanda, and the UN has sent in troops to help control the violence and protect the local people. Because the LRA has been less active around Assa, the Azande had thought they would be returning home soon, but this new development may keep them away. They must wait and see, as we all must.

Uncertainty is the root of what makes these people seem inaccessible. For our missions to the CAR, it began in 2011, with the sudden uncertainty of whether we would be able to get into the country. In January 2012, it was the uncertainty of the conditions we would find when we arrived there, of what equipment might be present other than what we carried in with us, of the friends we would see or who might be missing. And in June 2012, it was the uncertainty of whether we would be able to make it from Zemio to Obo given the availability of transportation, conditions on the path between the two villages, and the level of LRA activity in the area.

Despite the uncertainty, though, these missions to heal are life-changing events—for the many people we treat, for the local workers we train, and for the participants, who are never again able to look at their world in quite the same way.

This is the story of one of those life-changing missions: June 2012 in the Central African Republic.

PART I

TOWARD THE POLE— INTO THE CENTRAL AFRICAN REPUBLIC

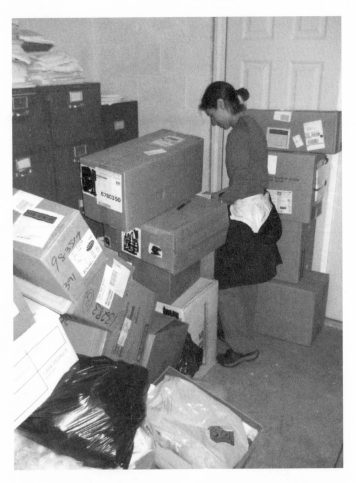

Claudia works to organize the donated and scavenged supplies into fourteen cargo bags during the Derwood, Maryland, packing party.

CHAPTER ONE

THE TEAM GATHERS

June 1–2, 2012, Derwood, Maryland, to Addis Ababa, Ethiopia

THROUGH SOME COMBINATION OF MINOR MIRACLES, WE WERE ALL seated in a Boeing 777, seven across, on an Ethiopian Airlines flight from Washington Dulles International Airport to Addis Ababa, Ethiopia. After a brief layover there, we were on to Entebbe, Uganda. And from there, it was on to the African pole of inaccessibility, in the Central African Republic (CAR).

Our group had gathered from several compass points just the day before, amid a downpour and tornado warnings, in Derwood, Maryland. The day had started with an early trip—at 6:50 a.m.—out to Dulles to pick up Claudia Vazquez. She is petite in stature at just ninety pounds, but has voluminous energy and enthusiasm. She is a veteran mission team member, and it showed in her well-packed bags; she understood that space on the trip came at a premium. A registered nurse (RN) and certified surgical first assistant (CFA), she had coordinated the vast number of various clinical kits for this trip after operating with me for the second time in South Sudan just six months before.

Under threat of a rainstorm, I drove Claudia to the National Mall so she could tour the newer monuments and then scurried over to George Washington University (GWU) to perform some eleventh-hour administrative tasks. Then we headed out to Derwood, phoning the others, who were flying into Baltimore and Reagan National Airports.

Dan Vryhof, another mission veteran, took the Metrorail to Derwood. He had flown in from Michigan, but he knew DC well after his previous orientation trips. He had just graduated from Calvin College in Grand Rapids, but he was preparing for his first year at GWU's medical school. He would enter with more time in an operating room than most of his colleagues would see in their first three years—this was his second medical mission with me in just six months. And with Dan on the trip, I knew I would have at least one running partner—if we found any time to run.

Dan first contacted me after he heard me speak at Calvin College, my alma mater, in January 2011. (A podcast of the speech, "Mission to Heal," is available on iTunes.) In his email, he had described his earnest wish to do what I do, where I do it, and had told me about his interest in applying to medical school. Since hearing my lecture and noting my affiliation with George Washington University, he had moved GWU to the top of his application list. He asked to meet me when he came to DC to interview at the university. I responded and asked if he was related to Wesley Vryhof, who had taught me physics in high school. He responded, "Yes, and my grandfather said you were a very bright kid."

The Grand Rapids community is a small, tight-knit one.

In January 2012, one year after hearing me speak, Dan had accompanied me to South Sudan, Chad, and the CAR, just five months before our current trip. In April 2012, he attended the annual Students for Medical Missions Symposium at the University of Toledo, where my student teams present on their experiences. Dan's brother Nick, friend Josh VanderWall, and junior classmate Kyle Burghgraef came with him. At this conference, which is held in association with the induction ceremonies of the Medical Mission Hall of Fame Foundation, Josh asked me if he could join us on the June return trip to the CAR, and both Nick and Kyle asked to be included on the missions planned for January 2013. They would be part of a half dozen Calvin College premed students signed up for missions with me to Nigeria, South Sudan, and two islands of the Philippines, along with students from other schools.

Dan and Nick's father, Steven Vryhof, met me when he accompanied Dan to DC, and on that trip he had asked to become an active part of my ongoing mission efforts. He is now a crucial member of the M2H board of directors.

Three generations of Vryhofs have subsequently visited me in Derwood, and by coincidence, Dan's grandparents, Wes and Fran, are close friends of my sister, Shirley, and she had already shared with them the audiotapes, narrative texts, and photojournalism I regularly send home from these remote missions.

I picked Dan up at the Shady Grove metro station, along with Bruce Visniski, a CFA from Muskegon, Michigan. This was Bruce's first trip with me, though he'd long wanted to go on one. He had first read about the missions on the National Institute of First Assisting (NIFA) website, where the CEO, Jerry Kekos, recommended the experience and explained that NIFA would help by covering some of the travel expenses. Bruce is also a hunter and had recently discovered an avid pupil in his seventeen-year-old daughter, Jenna.

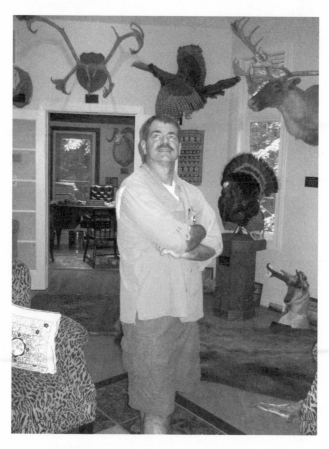

Bruce gets his chance to scope out the Derwood game room.

Dan's friend Josh VanderWall arrived soon after. He grew up on a farm in Marne, Michigan, and is entering Michigan State University's College of Human Medicine in Grand Rapids, Michigan. (This school was opened in 2010, and in May 2014, I'll be its inaugural commencement speaker.) Josh and Dan could almost be twins—they are both about six feet tall with short sandy hair and blue eyes—and they look especially similar when both are wearing their blue Mission to Heal T-shirts. Josh, like Bruce, is a hunter.

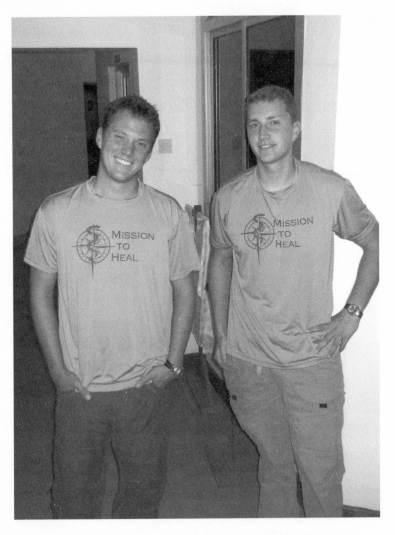

Dan and Josh look almost like twins, especially in their Mission to Heal T-shirts.

If I can help it, I never go on a medical mission alone. I have always brought medical students and other health-care workers who are interested in learning from and educating others. (The exception is when I travel to areas of active warfare.) The purpose is to educate both ways; I want the students and team members to learn from those who have never been in school or a developed medical setting, to see what care is possible using only eyes and fingers and ears. And I want the indigenous workers to recognize that those accompanying me are young folk who are at the same level in terms of their knowledge but who are accomplishing great things by dint of diligent effort and applied discipline. I want everyone involved to see that we are all in the process of learning.

It was beginning to seem that I had constructed the group for this mission around two of my passions: running and hunting. Of course, that wasn't quite the case. Only those who are prepared to pull their weight in a surgical setting need apply. Although, on this trip, we would have one additional member, which was a bit of a sore spot for me. But I'll get to that in a moment.

In the mission control room—my basement—Claudia had set to work organizing the drugs and surgical kits into the fourteen bags that would hold all of our supplies and belongings. (At the time, there was no additional charge for two checked bags per person. Now it costs $70 to $100 per bag after the first.) The supplies had been primarily scrounged from overstocks at local hospitals, the Medical Mission Hall of Fame Foundation's distribution center, and Project SAVE (Salvage All Valuable Equipment). The other team members helped Claudia while I ran through the orientation for the mission, talked about expectations, and passed around the photo album from our January trip. The pictures of Flore got much attention as we waited for word from the last two team members, who were on planes that were trying to land in stormy conditions.

Leenta Nel, a CFA originally from South Africa who now lives in Victoria, British Columbia, wouldn't arrive at Dulles until after midnight, so she would spend the night at a hotel near the airport and meet us at the terminal in the morning. Like Bruce, Leenta was a newbie and had heard about M2H through the NIFA website. Despite the fact that she was caring for her ailing mother and her own family, she had long-held hopes of returning to Africa to serve. She read *Gifts from the Poor* (Austin, Texas: Greenleaf Book Group Press, 2011), decided that she and I were kinfolk, and signed up for the next mission.

The last to arrive was our lone ranger, Joseph Chavez—the sticking point I referred to earlier. Despite delays, he landed in Baltimore and found a van to get him to Derwood, where he arrived at 2:30 in the morning. Dan and I welcomed him in the wet driveway despite the fact that we would be leaving for the airport in just four hours. And we discovered that our work wasn't yet over. Joe had been misinformed and brought along a large backpack that would need to be checked. We would have to leave behind one of the fourteen big, blue bags we had loaded with cataract kits and other surgical supplies. Joe was the odd man out of our highly motivated group, through no fault of his. He was simply someone I did not know, had not vetted, and had not invited on the mission, but who had been offered an all-expense-paid trip—funded by me—by an overreaching administrator who wanted to do a documentary of our work abroad. The trouble was, Joe had never traveled outside of the country, had never been in an operating room, had no experience filming medical procedures or travelogues, and had never shot or produced a documentary. And we had no contract for a specific work product. But it was done, he was going (a nonrefundable ticket had already been purchased), and I could only hope for the best and focus on the work in front of us.

Most of us understood the difficulties that lay ahead, but the excitement of the team was palpable. One encouraging point was Flore. Dan had seen her firsthand, and the rest of the team had seen her photos and learned what we had done.

Six months before, we had arrived with her, her brother, Blaise, and her caregiver, Ambroise, in Kijabe, Kenya, with the hope of saving her life. First, though, we had to get past the somewhat ridiculous hurdle of immigrating into Kenya. We stood in line in front of a Kenyan woman in a cage-like booth while Flore sat on a baggage cart nearby, feeling sick from the long flight and still covering her face with her scarf. Despite her hideous facial deformity and the turmoil of trying to get out of the country and provide for her children on short notice, she sat calmly on a baggage cart with her neatly painted toenails poking through her sandals.

We handed the woman our passports and visas and she quickly responded, "You do us a disservice. You must pay for a new visa. We must have a $100 bill."

"Here it says multi-entry visa," I said. "This is only our second entry. And this visa is good for five more months."

"No," she said. "You must pay me $100 now."

I was exhausted and worried about Flore and rapidly losing my patience. There was no way I was going to pay this woman $100—money that would go into her pocket, not the till—because each of the others with me would also have to pay $100, and none of us had it. I looked up and saw a sign on her booth: "Anti-Corruption Police: If you encounter any corruption, you are to notify this number."

"Where are the police?" I asked.

"Well, you will have to go downtown and notify there." Of course, we would have to immigrate first and then pay another $100 to get downtown, but neither of those points mattered. It was 5:30 p.m. on a Friday and the offices were closed.

Dan, who is generally a soft-spoken guy, stepped up and got in this woman's face. "Look, you fool," he said, "we have paid and we're not going to pay twice." Then Jon Hildebrandt got involved and began yelling at the woman in Kiswahili. All during this circus, I had my arm around Flore's shoulders, rocking her back and forth.

Finally, I decided to end the commotion. I stood up and said to the woman, "Look, you've got your thing, and I've got mine," and then pushed Flore on the baggage cart through the gate, with the rest of the team following me. The woman blustered at us, but what could she do? Call the police because we weren't letting her steal from us?

We went out into the parking lot, collected our bags, and I negotiated a taxi to carry Flore, Ambroise, and Blaise to the neighborhood around Kijabe Hospital, several hours to the west on the scarp of the Great Rift Valley. I had written a thorough letter of referral for Flore, emphasizing that she was not beyond the bounds of resectability and listing all of my credentials and affiliations to help ensure she got care. Flore, Ambroise, and Blaise also needed money to live, so I gave them $500, and Scott Downing, a missionary kid (MK) who'd been born in Africa when his parents had worked in Assa Congo with AIM and who was with us on the mission as a "homecoming" to his Azande friends now in CAR, gave them another couple hundred dollars.

As the rest of the team prepared to return home, flying west through Europe, I prepared for my departure east to Doha, Qatar. From there I would fly to the Philippines, where I would be on another adventure doing similar surgical missions on the Asian extension of this circumnavigation. But Flore, Ambroise, and Blaise were on their own adventure. They had arrived in an unknown place and had to find a place to stay, which turned out to be a sort of flophouse that the three of them moved into. The next morning, a Saturday, they went over to the hospital and found a woman named Susan, a plastic surgery resident visiting from Vanderbilt University Medical Center in Nashville, Tennessee. Fortuitously, Susan had been a resident of John Tarpley's; Tarpley and I were both fellows at the National Cancer Institute. When she saw my affiliations, she emailed him, and he responded that I wasn't a fly-by-night surgeon or a tourist on a pleasure trip, that this is my life's work, and that if I said the tumor was resectable, they should have a go at it.

Sometimes, where you've been and who you know make a difference. Two days later, Flore had her operation done—masterfully.

With James Umweke's knock on the door at 6:30 a.m., we all rendezvoused in the drive, scrambling to eat the perishables from the refrigerator as we loaded our bags into the back of a Ford F-250. James is a member of the Ibo tribe and was born in Ozu Abam, a small village in Abia Province, Nigeria. He came to America and became a civil engineer (he now works for the Maryland Department of Transportation). James found me through the mysterious web of people who operate humanitarian missions. Janice Walker of Project SAVE called me one day from Chico, California, to tell me that an African fellow was trying to build a clinic in his home village and had asked her for a container of supplies. (Janice tells me I'm the only recipient of her excellent equipment stock who ever returns to give presentations on the good works that their efforts make possible.) The man, James, had family and other connections on the scene who would help him do the right thing with the shipment, despite the notorious graft in Nigeria. So I set up a meeting with James at Derwood (telling him to bring his running shoes, since I was going out for a ten kilometer run—in which James joined in and reported later to his wife that he had just performed the first run of his life!), and he has been a most valuable ally ever since, helping me with M2H presentations and fund-raisers. In December, we would be going to Nigeria for the opening of his clinic.

The pickup truck belongs to John McLaurin, our new M2H board chairman. He is also a vice president of Safari Club International (SCI), an organization dedicated to promoting wildlife conservation worldwide and to protecting the freedom to hunt. As an attorney with an office in the Pentagon, John had been invaluable in helping us through a recent reorganization and discovered along the way that we were not a registered 501(c)(3) organization, as I had been told we were. Amateur errors in the administration of the organizational component of M2H, which I had entrusted to others, were the source of the problem. SCI also loaned us the giant, blue duffel bags for carting our supplies and backpacks.

The excitement of pulling together a miraculous team for what we hoped would be an exceptional mission was suddenly clouded as we climbed into vehicles to head to Dulles. James handed me his phone, displaying an excoriating email he had received from one of the supporters of M2H. The man's son, a volunteer firefighter, had accompanied us on a previous mission to

South Sudan and then began doing work for M2H, but it had not gone well. I had to censure him for overreaching his authority and committing the organization and its resources (read: my resources) to high-liability and high-cost deals—without discussing it with me. He was the one who had offered the trip to Joe. He had also designated himself as cofounder of M2H and had stripped the endowment.

It takes more than eager enthusiasm to help and money donated from some anonymous source to launch a medical mission into a remote site. Most don't realize that the organization is formed around my credentials, experience, medical licenses, and my financial support. Most of the mission participants cover their airfare, and we use donated surgical supplies, but each mission costs my account somewhere between $35,000 and $50,000. Still, that is how it seems it must be: If we were beholden to other nongovernmental organizations (NGOs), we would not be able to do the work we do in the places we do it—helping populations that most people believe, or want to believe, are inaccessible. Every action would have to be cleared by a central board, and every time we entered a country we would have to ask permission from the government to do the work. Instead, we operate without drag and avoid political negotiations by playing the simple role of visiting physicians.

Official international agencies like the UN, or multilateral, governmental, or nongovernmental organizations have layers and layers of constraints on their ability to help oppressed peoples. To go into an area to assist displaced and refugee peoples, who are often starving and sick, they must receive a request or invitation and be permitted by the sovereign state to work within its borders. Such permission is often given, sometimes reluctantly, by a "host government" that bargains for equal or better treatment for its own equally poor citizens, with considerable skimming for wealthy elites. To have refugee populations, often of the same ethnic group, inside walled-off camps with access to food, education, and health care creates tension with the citizens of the host country. As nonrefugees, they have no access to such aid, despite the fact that they have similar needs.

The disgruntled and impoverished Turkana people of the deserts near Lokichoggio, Kenya, lived adjacent to the Kakuma refugee camp, where the South Sudanese "Lost Boys" and a few girls were being taught English and job skills and were supplied with food, clothing, health care, and even resettlement options that included airfare to Australia, Canada, and the United States. The Turkana demanded of me, "How do I get into one of these camps next to where I have lived my whole life? No one has ever come to help me or given me any aid!" Flore represented an extreme case of special services not accessible to most people in Kijabe, Kenya, where she was treated. As part of the needy host-country population, the people of Kijabe do not have an advocate or sponsor of the kind Flore had attracted due to the extremity of her need.

This difference is a crucial reason that some NGOs are limited in the aid they can offer to certain persecuted populations. Generally, they have to follow the rules of refugees, which means that until a group of people crosses an international border—until they transform from internally displaced persons (IDPs) to refugees—they often cannot be helped. If the sovereign state is the persecutor, it won't likely invite or grant permission to outsiders who want to help. The number of persecuted peoples who have not been so fortunate as to make it across an international border, many of whom were repulsed by effective border security, is higher than the refugee populations. Yet these IDPs are no less needy. I have not been invited by Sudan's President Bashir to help the people of Darfur, whom he has been strafing, earning him an indictment from the International Criminal Court. I had not been invited by the Burmese military junta (of Myanmar) to help the Karen and Shan peoples, whom they have been persecuting. But I am not obligated to wait for such an unlikely invitation. Chad's porous eastern border with Darfur is not so impenetrable that a small group cannot later request forgiveness for its unsophisticated ignorance of an arbitrary boundary. The Salween River is not so wide as to prevent my entry into Burma from Thailand as freight. Tell whatever CAR government survives the most recent coup that I am very sorry, that my focus upon medical care and patient well-being has rendered me border-blind, as I hotly pursue a patient constituency that has been moved around time and again ahead of many hostile forces.

Of course, I am often limited, too. I had first wanted to go into the DRC to help the Assa IDPs when they fled into the bush, but I could not enter the country in that situation, even to find, let alone help, them. I would have had to fly to the CAR, through its distant capital at Bangui, and then cross the border, which would have been an incursion into a sovereign state, an entry into a hostile DRC without official immigration. And getting caught doing something like that would limit my later effectiveness in the region.

In addition to my licenses and certifications in the United States, I have spent time and resources to obtain medical licenses to practice in such places as Nigeria and South Sudan, and that covers much of the work I do and the work of the students who accompany me. These licenses also allow me to delegate to and "certify" indigenous operators to work independently in very limited ways once I have trained them.

But now, thanks to the indiscretions of the overreaching administrator who had, among other things, offered the free trip to Joseph Chavez, M2H was operating in a deficit, and it would be my responsibility to pull us out of it. I couldn't rescind the promises for supplies and clinical care this volunteer had made. I had asked him to stay on without the authority to commit resources, but once he had been censured he took his baseball bat and went home, smashing windows along the way. His father's email stated that the family wanted nothing further to do with M2H, just when we needed fundraising support to rebuild the endowment.

It was awkward to be battling a rear-guard political and diplomatic fire while trying to press ahead with qualified people on a mission to help those in need in one of the most remote places on earth. But of course, that is what we did.

Having arrived at Dulles, we met Leenta, and the seven of us began the magical balancing act of getting all our checked bags tagged and weighed in at fifty pounds, and all our carry-on bags weighed in at twenty pounds. With a little sleight of hand that involved shifting small items from one bag to another after weighing, the balance was finally cleared. Joe shot a video of my send-off talk, and we departed on an adventure that would no doubt change each of us in some fundamental way.

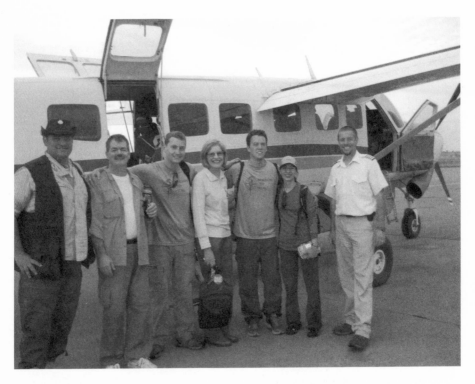

The fantastic team, as well as our trusty pilot, Jon Hildebrandt, by the Cessna 208 Caravan that would transport us across two countries to Zemio, CAR.

CHAPTER TWO

THE OTHER SIDE OF THE WORLD

June 3–4, 2012, Addis Ababa, Ethiopia, to Uganda

WE WERE ZOMBIES, SITTING AT GATE 11 WAITING TO BOARD OUR flight to Entebbe, Uganda. I made a cursory attempt to get some Ethiopian stamps to send the few cards I had written on the flight, but it seemed that they would have to be sent from Entebbe after all—they couldn't be mailed from Addis Ababa unless we immigrated, and I was too wilted from the long flight to deal with the security hassles.

Despite the fact that it had been a thirteen-hour flight, on which we'd seen day, night, and day again, Dan and I had gotten little rest. Every time we began to fall asleep, a Cameroonian woman in the window seat would ask, "Why are you trying to sleep? Did you not go to bed last night?" And she needed to get up at least once an hour, which required us to get up too. Finally, I suggested that she would no doubt be more comfortable in the aisle seat, and I moved over to the window. So, Dan and I made it until 7:25 a.m., dawn over Addis Ababa, still awake.

I explained to the team that we had traveled back in time and it was now 2004. Ethiopia follows a unique calendar that is based on the ancient Gregorian and Coptic calendars—their years date about 7.5 behind the rest of the world, and the date changes at noon rather than midnight. When I was here in September 2007, I ran the Millennium Marathon, sponsored by Ethiopian Airlines, as the year changed from 1999 to 2000 at noon on September 11, 2007.

Joe was taking a few video clips as we moved from point to point and would film whenever I gave a brief orientation speech. It was a reminder of the administrative quagmire at home—but I couldn't focus on that when I was trying hard just to get us and our massive load of supplies to the most inaccessible place on the African continent.

I was sitting in my room in the Central Inn in Entebbe, trying to stay awake long enough for the power to come back on so I could take a shower. I thought it would be the last warm water any of us would see for weeks, when and if the power came back on in Entebbe. We would leave the next morning for the Central African Republic and Zemio, where water, let alone the temperature of it, would be a critical concern.

Our flight had arrived in Entebbe as planned. Uganda was a welcome sight, both because of the hotel bed that I knew was waiting and because of the beautiful surroundings. Winston Churchill labeled Uganda the "Pearl of Africa" for a reason.

Entebbe lies on a peninsula that juts into the greatest of the African Great Lakes—Lake Victoria. It is the second-largest freshwater lake in the world, behind Lake Superior. (The lake containing the largest amount of freshwater, because its depth is so great, is Lake Baikal in Siberia.) Just to the north sits Kampala, the capital of Uganda. The Entebbe International Airport—used by the military, NGOs, and commercial lines—sits at the end of the peninsula, where there is room for its long runways. Entebbe—in pro-Palestinian Uganda—was the site of the famous 1976 Israeli commando raid to rescue one hundred hostages off a hijacked Air France flight. I have been in and out of Entebbe many times since then, and the bullet holes have largely been patched up.

Entebbe is also one of the airports used by AIM AIR—Africa Inland Mission's air support, which transports medical, relief, and missionary personnel and supplies, sometimes even acting as medevac. (AIM AIR is the primary organization I charter planes from in central Africa; I have been flying with them for several generations of pilots, many of whom are missionary kids whose parents I worked with at the mission stations.) One special reason we had chartered them for this mission was that AIM AIR has an exclusive agreement with the government of the Central African Republic that allows them to immigrate and emigrate through Zemio, on the southeast border, rather than first flying to the capital, Bangui—six barrels of Jet A-1 fuel and $14,000 to the west—to immigrate officially before traveling within the country.

I have had a long relationship with AIM, chartering their aircraft, staying in their mission houses, befriending their local missionaries. I pay for the services I receive—for every person on every flight, and for every night's stay and every meal at the mission stations—but ours has been a friendly partnership for years and I admire the work of the many missionaries with the organization.

At the Entebbe airport, a fellow by the name of Deo from the Central Inn was to greet us by holding up a sign: "Dr. Grand Geelhoed." We only saw the sign much later, though, as we were busy immigrating into Uganda, exchanging currency, collecting fourteen bags and attempting to check them into the AIM AIR hangar, and trying to buy phone cards for those who had smartphones so they would work at least while we were in Entebbe. Amazingly, I had heard that there was a new cell tower near the approach to the dirt airstrip in Zemio, so we were trying to determine whether these phone cards might work there. If they did, it would be a miracle of modern communication.

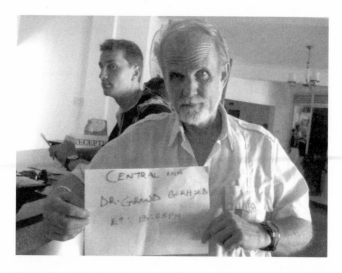

The sign Deo of the Central Inn was holding, a call for Dr. "Grand" Geelhoed.

The AIM hangar and offices were closed, so we went to the information center to find somebody to open them for us. A woman named Lydia at the information desk found a fellow named Hassan in her contacts and gave us his information. We got Leenta's new phone card working and called him, and he said he was a contractor for AIM. Hassan could be induced to come to the airport to open the office and store the bags—if I would give him money for fuel. The other members of the team remained with the bags inside the sterile zone of the airport behind armed guards while I ventured out to meet Hassan. When he arrived, I gave him a $20 bill, but he returned it and asked for another. There was a small nick in the upper corner of the first one, he pointed out, so I replaced it with another of my crisper bills. With negotiations complete, we stashed the bags in an office with the trolleys.

We finally reached Ron Pontier, an AIM pilot stationed at Entebbe, but discovered that he would not be flying us out the next day. Instead, Jon Hildebrandt would be making an unusual Sunday flight in the Cessna. I was happy to learn that Jon would be returning to the CAR with us. We would have to be up at five, out after a six o'clock breakfast for a seven o'clock wheels-up. In the meantime, we needed to get to the Central Inn, gather some last-minute supplies, and rest.

As we were talking with Ron, Deo found us—or rather, I finally saw the sign he was holding outside the airport. Unfortunately, once we arrived at the Central Inn, we discovered more hurdles to be leapt. Our four rooms cost about what a US hotel would charge for one room. However, the power was out, the machine could not read my credit card, and when the electricity eventually came on, I was told that I couldn't access my Mission to Heal bank account. I would just have to put the rooms on my American Express card. Easy—until they came back and said that the machine was not working. I responded with, "Well, it will go through when the power is restored." To which I was told that, no, the machine has never been working. The transaction, it turned out, required new, crisp US $100 bills. The signs announcing that credit cards were accepted is just window dressing for tourists. So I paid with some more of my precious cash.

In the meantime, Dan and Josh went out to buy a new kerosene stove, since we could not find the correct propane bottles for the stove we had. Of course, the right propane bottles could have been found in America, but no airline—at least none that we would want to travel with—was going to let us check them. The stove is critical: It is our only method of boiling water in a pressure cooker to sterilize our instruments and gowns. (Now, in retrospect since the events at the Boston Marathon in April 2013, what chance do you think I might have of boarding any airplane anywhere with my essential pressure cooker "autoclave"?)

That afternoon, we heard from Jon Hildebrandt, who would be arriving in Entebbe in the evening and would be ready to leave early tomorrow. I finally showered and unsuccessfully tried to access the wireless Internet in the Central Inn lobby—amid more power outages. When the television was operating, it only broadcast the Diamond Jubilee celebration for Queen Elizabeth II going on in London. At 7:00 p.m., the seven of us rendezvoused in the dining hall for a pasta dinner. Dan Vryhof successfully logged on to the Internet and I quickly sent a few of the notes of our arrival I had written on the airplane. By then, none of us could keep our eyes open.

Our new day started with a superb breakfast buffet, the best part of our Central Inn stay. By 6:30 a.m. we were on the shuttle to the airport. There we met Ron Pontier, who was taking his daughter back to school at the Rift Valley Academy. Our surgical kits had been transferred by Hassan and Jon Hildebrandt, who were waiting for us on the tarmac next to an Ilyushin Soviet-era airlifter with a large UN decal on its side. That wasn't the plane we would be taking, of course. AIM had a Cessna 208 Caravan, a small turboprop cargo plane with seating for nine or ten, depending on whether the last seat was removed to accommodate luggage. It could land on the small dirt airstrips where we were headed.

We once again tallied all the bag and body weight, this time for Hassan. I introduced the superb surgical team to Jon as we clambered aboard the Caravan. Then we turned the discussion to the logistics of the trips that would take us there and back again. We were heading toward the African pole of inaccessibility. Logistics were everything.

After delivering us to Zemio station, Jon or another AIM pilot would return in ten days ("más o menos") with the Cessna to either Zemio or Obo, depending on where we ended up on June 15. We hoped to travel from Zemio to Obo, but we wouldn't know if it would be possible until we were in Zemio. It was the rainy season, and while the two subprefectures were only about seventy miles apart, the "road" between them was little more than a rutted muddy path through the jungle. Add to that the fact that the senselessly violent Lord's Resistance Army (LRA) is active in the area, and we had an uncertain situation. Plus, a joint action of the African Union, primarily using Uganda People's Defence Force (UPDF) troops and AFRICOM for support, was in force in the area to try to rout the LRA, and because of this, we wouldn't just need to find vehicles to get us there, we would also need a security contingent. There was, however, a possibility that Mark Pearson, an honorary British consul (England does not have an embassy in the CAR), might broker air transport for us with the UPDF, which had planes in the area.

Given all of this, if we could make the trip overland to Obo, we wouldn't want to do it twice. AIM would be flying into the area to pick us up anyway, so it didn't particularly matter whether we were picked up in Zemio or Obo. By air, they were only thirty minutes apart. By land, it could take days. But we couldn't afford for a plane to fly all the way there simply to transport us in the middle of our trip. Much of the cargo capacity on the Cessna is taken up by the fuel it needs for the return trip, unless extra fuel has been flown in on previous trips and stored at Zemio. With each round trip flight costing about $12,000, that certainly wasn't an option.

We would have to wait, with fingers crossed, to find out whether traveling to Obo would be possible or worth the risk. Traveling slowly across the land was dangerous and used up time we could use to see patients.

This trip was very different from our previous two to the CAR. In January, just six months prior, we had chartered the AIM plane for the entire time we were in the CAR; it was only six days "on the ground" and cost less in fuel than chartering two round trips, one to fly us in and one to fly us out. On that trip, getting to Obo was as simple as a quick flight, within a much longer charter travel through South Sudan, Chad, and the CAR—the longest trip of Jon Hildebrandt's twenty-year flying career. This time, we would be in the CAR for almost two weeks, and one of AIM's planes couldn't sit idle on an airstrip that long.

Leenta asked if we would go to Obo or Zemio first, noting that Obo was closer. I corrected her, incorrectly as it turned out, and said that Zemio was seventy miles closer. But Leenta had looked at the map and seen that Obo is closer to Arua, our necessary last stop in Uganda. However, we were compelled to travel to Zemio first; it's the only point of entry available to us in the eastern part of the country. Even with our special dispensation to bypass entry through Bangui, we could only travel through the official alternative entrepôts of the unprepossessing airstrip at Zemio.

A year and a half before, in January 2011, we weren't struggling to move within the CAR, we were struggling in vain to get into the CAR. AIM's very precious permit to fly into Zemio had expired literally while we were in the air. Elections had just occurred, and as is often the case, the country's administration was in chaos. Elections in the CAR don't entail a smooth transition from one leadership to the next or continuity of the few government services that exist. In the capital, it was unclear who was now responsible for these permits.

In fits and starts, we had moved closer and closer to the CAR border, thanks to the UPDF hosting us at their airstrips in camps set up to support their hunt for Joseph Kony. We finally stalled at Nzara, in western South Sudan. Every day, we worked to find a way into the CAR that wouldn't require us spending an additional $14,000 in fuel. In between calls to everyone I knew and negotiations with a variety of organizations, including the US embassy, the UPDF, and others, we watched battery-powered reality TV broadcast by Al Jazeera, including *American Idol*! There was no work for us to do. We even got permission from certain organizations to fly into Obo with the UPDF, which was making frequent runs. But the Obo commander would not allow us on the helicopters, stating that he could face a court-martial if he did.

Meanwhile, Mark Pearson, in Bangui at the time, chased down one person after another, trying to get somebody to sign off on the permit. He spends much of his time in the eastern CAR and works closely with AIM. He understood the importance of the permits not only to our mission but also to the long-term goal of making this inaccessible region accessible. We could have spent the money and flown to Bangui and back again, but if we had, it could have set a precedent we'd be forced to stick to forever. We knew we had to protect AIM AIR's permit to travel in and out of Zemio.

After a useless week of waiting—with supplies and skills desperately needed in the CAR—for someone to be assigned to the role of FAA, we had to abort the mission and return home.

After her operation, getting Flore back to Obo presented similar difficulties. We couldn't afford the $12,000 to simply charter a flight for her, Ambroise, and Blaise, so we had to rely on a series of previously scheduled AIM flights and the charity of the pilots. Jon Hildebrandt and I corresponded back and forth to figure out how to get them from point A to point Z via points B through Y. They made it by road from Kijabe to Nairobi, the capital of Kenya, where they spent a night or two at the apartment of one of the AIM pilots while they looked for ground transportation from Nairobi to Lokichoggio (or just "Loki," to most) in northern Kenya. Once in Loki, they managed to catch an AIM AIR flight to Uganda. From Uganda, they took another road trip and then caught another AIM flight. Eventually, after days and days of travel—especially hard for a postoperative patient—they made it back to Zemio and Obo.

We took off from Entebbe in the Cessna. As we flew over the White Nile, we banked to circle a plume of water rising from thundering white, foamy falls. Murchison Falls, named after the president of the Royal Geographic Society in the 1860s, Sir Roderick Murchison, is a thrilling sight to behold from the air. We learned that Jon would be taking his family there on holiday the next week as he awaited the pickup of our team in either Zemio or Obo. I mentioned my long-held ambition to explore the falls and asked that he take good notes for my potential visit. We circled above so our amateur and professional photographers could shoot it.

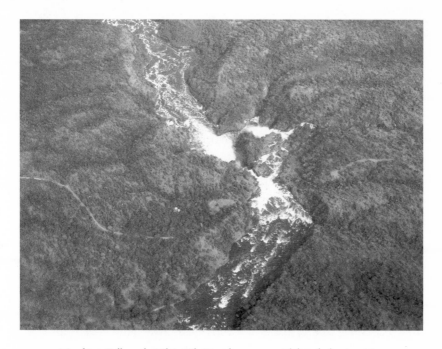

Murchison Falls on the White Nile River, long on my wish list of adventure trips.

I could imagine hippos floating in the downstream side at the fringes of whirlpools, and crocodiles lying on the shallow banks in the heavy spray of the rainy season. What looked like windblown laundry-soap foam settled along the trails of black water that followed the tumult of the churning chasm. We did not invade the restricted airspace over the falls, but we may have risked the ire of the park officials by buzzing at a still-respectful altitude as we looked on in awe. "Scenes so lovely must have been gazed upon by angels in their flight" was David Livingstone's response to a similar view of Victoria Falls over the Zambezi River. It was a fitting thought.

After the falls, we flew toward a bridge on the White Nile adjacent to a small town I had not seen before. The airspace around it was restricted as well, according to the flight mapping, and we guessed that it was near a presidential summer palace. The reelected president of Uganda is Yoweri Museveni, and his portrait can be seen on every wall at the Entebbe airport (though many would say he re-stole the presidency more than he re-won it). Almost every picture shows him in a rather ridiculous black Stetson hat. It makes him look a bit goofy, even innocent, but that is not an accurate impression. The revolt in the late 1980s that fueled the rebellion of the northern tribes of Uganda proved that. Despite the fact that he has been lauded for bringing stability and growth to a war-torn country since his rise to the presidency in 1986 and for helping to stem the tide of HIV/AIDS, his focus on southern Ugandan peoples and marginalization of the northern ethnic groups led to much opposition and the rise of Joseph Kony and the LRA in northern Uganda, South Sudan, the DRC, and the CAR.

Kony is power hungry, brutal, and deranged, so saying that Museveni may be better than Kony isn't saying much. For better or worse, Museveni is the recognized leader of Uganda, at least the more populous southern half. He was "duly elected"—by the half of the population that had a chance to vote, the half not actively shooting at him from the north. As is the case with most unsavory leaders, we have to take the situation as a political given and work with it as best we can. Unhappily, we are linked with Museveni. But the one rule of reality is change, now more than ever.

Given what we knew, we would not risk intercepting missiles by invading the president's protected airspace.

We landed in Arua, Uganda, to roll out the barrels—of Jet A-1 fuel. This was our last opportunity to refuel before the approximately five-hundred-mile, two-and-a-half-hour flight over the DRC to the border of the CAR, where Zemio sits. We have our own barrels of jet fuel spotted here, and we can take on two drums of fuel to give Jon enough endurance. In Zemio, he'll take on an additional barrel to get him back to Juba, South Sudan, where he lives.

Oddly, at the Arua airfield there was a large cornerstone dedicated to Mobutu Sese Seko, the former leader of what is now the Democratic Republic of the Congo, listing all of his titles, including "The All-Conquering Hero," "He Who Goes from Triumph to Triumph," and "Cock Among Hens." He is depicted in his well-known leopard-skin cap, which he alone, in all of the nation's population, was allowed to wear. Mobutu came into power as president in 1967 after leading two coups in what was then Zaire. He was deposed in 1997 after a corrupt, iron-fisted, thirty-year rule marked by nepotism and embezzlement.

Ironically, only here in Uganda, a nation that wasn't the one he led and exploited, would you find a cornerstone dedicated to the dead despot Mobutu. And it was even more odd because Uganda's Museveni had partnered with Paul Kagame, then Rwanda's minister of defence, to lead a group of regional government forces and local opposition groups in Zaire (now the DRC) to overthrow Mobutu. They had taken action after Mobutu issued an order evicting all ethnic Tutsis from the country, on penalty of death. The action was over quickly. Mobutu's army fell before the marching forces because their only experience was in suppression of unarmed citizens—they had no knowledge of how to defend their country from armed rebels or foreign invaders.

As ever in my travels, *sic transit gloria mundi*—thus passes the glory of the world.

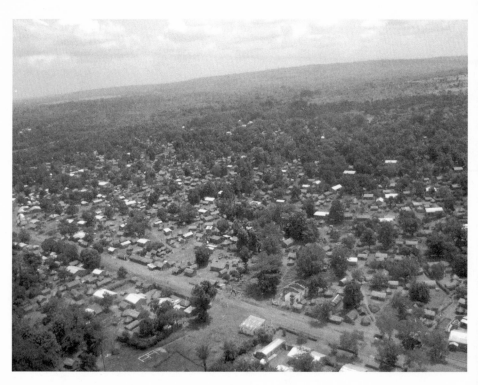

A beautiful view of Zemio, the thatch- and metal-roofed buildings surrounded by the equatorial forest.

CHAPTER THREE

ENTEBBE TO ZEMIO

June 4, 2012, Zemio, Central African Republic

WE SWOOPED DOWN OVER THE BORDER BETWEEN THE CENTRAL African Republic and the Democratic Republic of the Congo, flying over the Mbomou River. Crossing this river to evade the Lord's Resistance Army (LRA) had turned the Azande of Assa, DRC, into refugees.

Our entry into the CAR required two landings, first in the town of Zemio and then in the village of the Zemio mission station. In the town of Zemio, we have to immigrate officially with our $200 visas. As we approached the airstrip, the Australian-accented female voice of the TAWS—the terrain awareness and warning system—sounded throughout the cabin: "Pull up! Pull up!" The pilot usually mutes this warning as an airplane approaches landing, since one is expected to get well below five hundred feet in order to land, but the echoing calls to awaken the pilot were less than assuring to the passengers, who heard panic in the TAWS voice. I tried to explain that the alarm call was necessary on the low approach to the laterite airstrip, made muddy by the rainy season. Over the drone of the engine, my reassurance, incompletely understood, might have been as unsettling as the call of the TAWS.

Zemio is the remotest and smallest airfield on which some in the plane had ever landed. It is the last outpost of the CAR government; they likely put the airfield here because of the mission stations in the area and the number of expatriates coming in and out of this region.

"I still can't believe I'm here!" Bruce exclaimed.

Ambroise Soungouza, director of the Zemio clinic and one of the primary operators there, met us at the end of the airstrip and disappeared into an "official" hut, where the collected passports were duly admired. I had been corresponding with Ambroise, who speaks Pazande, French, and a bit of English, for years, but I had met him for the first time just six months before. As a member of the Zande tribe, he has a keen interest in trying to establish a greater number of fully functional clinics in the area. He returned shortly with the passports and joined us to become a passenger on the three-minute flight from Zemio to the Zemio mission station, about five miles away.

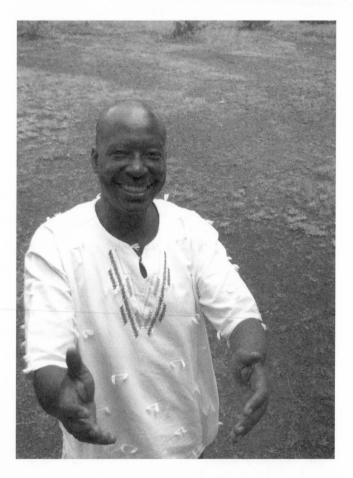

Ambroise Soungousa welcomes us at Zemio airstrip.

The stop at the town of Zemio is necessary because we have to immigrate there before we get all our supplies to the clinic at the mission station. On the way out, it's often necessary to load up the plane and then have the passengers meet it at the Zemio airfield for official emigration and takeoff— the airstrip at the mission station isn't long enough for the plane to take off fully loaded with fuel, cargo, and people. On our last trip, we had put Flore in the plane and then a few of the team members and I had traveled to Zemio on motorbikes.

We dipped low at the river and flew over the wide variety of trees in the tropical forest below, including the mango trees half in bloom and half in fruit (defining a monecious, "in one house" tree, containing both sexes in one tree, but with the maturation of each side of the tree on different timing so that the tree is not self-fertilizing), and then came down for a typically smooth Hildebrandt landing, despite a crosswind. As we came to the dogleg turn at the end of the even-shorter-than-the-last airstrip, I saw a man I knew immediately as Les Harris, though I had never met him.

Les and Mary Anne Harris have been working among the Azande for decades. When I was introducing the team and reported that Joe had recently created a video of the military ball on the *Queen Mary* at Long Beach, Les burst out, "Oh, we came across on the *Queen Mary's* last voyage, just before it was decommissioned!" The wonderful coincidence of their presence here is a perfect synergy. Les and Mary Anne had come from St. Petersburg, Florida, out of retirement with AIM, after having worked for decades in the same Congolese environments that I had. They had returned in 1967 as adults, but they had grown up in this region as MKs—missionary kids—and first met when they were barely more than toddlers. MKs often marry within their group—having grown up in the unique African environment, they have an "otherworldly" perspective that can be hard to explain to a potential spouse who doesn't share their background. MKs grow up in adjacent stations and inevitably are together at boarding school. They share language, culture, cuisine, and a lifestyle that revolves more around riding piki-pikis through the bush trails and shooting Cape buffalo than around senior proms and date nights at the movies. The AIM community is tightly-knit throughout the lives of missionaries. Les and Mary Anne are in the same AIM retirement community as Jon Hildebrandt's parents; Jon's father was the former director of AIM operations in Kenya.

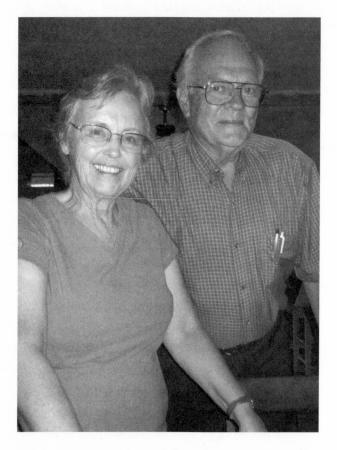

Our gracious hosts and frequent translators, Les and Mary Anne Harris.

The church is the centerpiece of the Zemio mission station, which, like similar stations in central Africa, was formerly supported by white missionaries who came to spread the Word and brought along a few accoutrements of modernity, including health care. AIM supported missions in all of Zande land—the northern Congo, the eastern CAR, South Sudan, a part of Uganda, and even a fringe of Chad. But its goal has been to "indigenize" the church; accordingly AIM has formed the Africa Inland Church, with branches for each country. The indigenization at Zemio and Obo has been completed, which is why the presence of Mary Anne and Les Harris was somewhat unusual—foreign missionaries are being extracted. Wendy Atkins, the most recent AIM worker in the area, had done amazing work through the mission to bring resources and attention to the refugee populations here. She and I had corresponded for three or four years, and she was the one who was standing by, anxious for our arrival, when we had been stuck in South Sudan, unable to enter the country. I have never met her, and now possibly never will, as I have heard that she is not likely returning to the CAR. AIM extracted most of its remaining missionaries in the area in the past year, partially due to the threat of violence.

That means that the Zemio station, like the Obo station, will be very much on its own. It will be left with the programs, the organization, and the structures of earlier AIM "urban planning," but AIM began building missions in the CAR back in the 1920s. Ninety years of dependence is hard to unravel.

Zemio, like other stations in the area, is well situated, this one on a bluff overlooking the Mbomou River valley. Everything is green and variegated in tropical splendor, except the cluster of well-built, ninety-year-old burned-brick houses. Tree-lined boulevards serve as walking paths to the different parts of the station and the two primary refugee camps that sit between the station and the town of Zemio, one filled with Azande from Assa.

Upon arrival, we were immediately surrounded by friends from Assa—with Jean Marco front and center. On the many trips I made to Assa, Jean Marco became my friend and my hunting guide, a man with much more skill than I when it came to providing meat for the village. His father, Bule, had been a much-relied-upon leader in the community, the go-to for everything from blacksmithing to hunting to drum carving; he had carved the massive talking drum used to send communiqués between villages. His name was ironic in the extreme—*bule* means "useless" in Kiswahili. Jean Marco's given name, Pung Balete, is almost as funny, a story I first told in *Out of Assa: Heart of the Congo* (Three Hawks Publishing, 2000). Zande tradition dictates that grandparents name the children in their families. Bule's wife was fairly well along in years when she became pregnant with Jean Marco, and when she gave birth, Bule traveled to deliver the good news to his parents in person—one of Assa's eldest and least fertile wives had just delivered a healthy son. When Bule's father heard, he blurted out *"Pung balete!"* which means, literally, "there is nothing in my mouth" and loosely "I am speechless." It became the new baby's name.

I had helped sponsor Jean Marco's children in their schooling, and I was particularly interested in helping his daughters in their studies to become nurses. The two girls study at Isiro, the closest thing to a city in the northeast DRC. After our wasted week in 2011, I had at least been able to send a care package in when we flew out of Nzara with Jon Hildebrandt and had transferred funds to Jean Marco through AIM pilot Ron Pontier at Entebbe, Uganda. Curiously, while many of the personal items (like a signed copy of *Out of Assa: Heart of the Congo*) I had sent through did not make it, the cash did, the exact opposite of what I expected.

While I have been happy to contribute to the girls' education, I have been concerned at times for Jean Marco and his family. I have seen the sometimes devastating, possibly lethal effects of what in Australia they call the "tall poppy syndrome." Leaving the village, becoming educated, and picking up skills that are not shared by the other indigenous people generates envy, and those who exhibit their merit are cut down to prove they are no better than others of the same origin. The powerful social lesson? Remain true to tribe rules and mores. There was once a young man in Assa who exhibited intellect and potential, so AIM sponsored him to study abroad so he could return and improve the conditions of the Azande. Unfortunately, when he returned, there were multiple attempts on his life and he eventually had to leave the village. He almost died during a visit from an uncle, and he did eventually die under mysterious circumstances. His wife and children now live in Atlanta, Georgia. I'm not certain they could ever safely return, even if they wanted to. People don't overachieve here without having to hire a private army to protect themselves from the envy of their own kind.

Despite the danger, Jean Marco has taken the ingenuity and other positive characteristics he inherited from his father to a higher level, working to organize and meet the needs of the Assa community. He has become invaluable to them. He was the one who led the families into the bush, and from there, across the river into the CAR. I offered prayers of thanks when I heard he had survived the trip to this region with the rest of the refugees, and when I saw him on our last trip, for the first time in fourteen years, I was elated.

I posed with Ambroise and Isaiah, the other operator and administrator of the clinic, for the first photographs Joe took in our new environment—well, new to some. Little Zande kids fought each other over the privilege of toting our many bags. Most of the bags went to the operating theater, and the couple containing clothing and personal items were carried off as the team members scattered to their quarters. I was returned to the same bed I had had on the last mission, in the main house with Leenta, Claudia, and the Harrises. We would be eating our meals here as well.

We adjourned for lunch and "getting to know you" time, finishing with a dessert of the sweetest and freshest pineapples ("anana" as they seem to be known by their French name everywhere except the USA)—the fruits were gifts from the population, and they are given to the Harrises so frequently that they often spoil. We had a number of volunteers willing to ensure that didn't happen. I introduced Ambroise, who was reluctant to try to say anything in English in front of an audience and a video camera, but he spoke about what we had done already with the clinic and produced his signed "certification of competence," which I had written up after our last trip in to operate with him in January.

Before the first attempted trip to the CAR, I had emailed Ambroise and asked him to obtain a certificate for me that stipulated that I could operate in the country. My licenses in Nigeria and South Sudan wouldn't necessarily carry over here. His response was essentially "Why would you need a certificate? I want *you* to certify *me*. There's no agency here that qualifies anybody to do anything, so if you want to come, do it."

Ambroise was uncomfortable for another reason: Our time was short. We would be doing consultations in the afternoon, and he knew there would be scores to see before dark—our usual time to retire from the fray. So we left to divide our personnel into teams, unpack the bags, and organize the stocks into medical kits to be left in the clinic's pharmacy and surgical kits for the OR, with further subdivision by procedure.

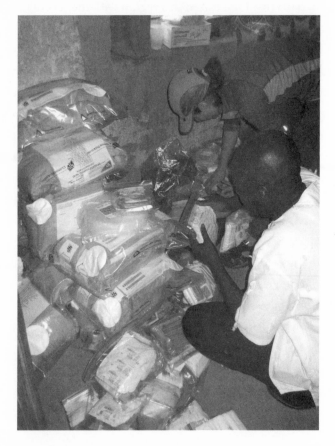

Claudia and Ambroise sort through our supplies and prepare for our opening day.

Then it was time to do consultations—as many as possible, as rapidly as we could.

Our trip in January had been successful in better supplying and organizing the Zemio clinic for a broader range of operations. Ambroise and Isaiah had grouped the patient information into four folders: "Goitre," "Hernie,"

"Gynecology and Myoma," and "Divers," which I assumed meant miscella-neous. In the intervening six months, they had been collecting patients for us to treat during this visit, which meant that on this trip, I didn't have to be my own referring physician, at least not for every patient. In January, we had seen hundreds of people in both Zemio and Obo, trying to squeeze them in while also doing as many operations as possible and taking the time to care-fully teach them to Ambroise and Isaiah. I had hoped that this trip might be slightly less hectic. The extra time in each village would help.

The patients they referred to me might have been skewed more toward the interests of the practitioners than to the most prevalent problems, but that seems somewhat unavoidable. Even in my early work in Assa, I treated far more goiters than other ailments because people knew of my interest in thyroid disease. Some of the procedures were the types of simpler operations I could train Ambroise and Isaiah to do. The third operator is Emmanuel, who typically assists; however, we hoped to have him independently do a few hernias, considerably stretching his portfolio. The role of the clinical officer, a nonphysician with on-the-job training, is a necessity here. Near poles of inaccessibility, we have to do whatever works, and training members of local tribes—Isaiah and Ambroise are both from the eastern CAR—to run local clinics works. Our goal is always to upgrade their skills.

Isaiah had had a six-week course that qualified him to operate indepen-dently on inguinal hernias, which occur when the lining of the abdominal cavity protrudes into the inguinal canal, a passage in the abdominal wall where the round ligament exists in women and the spermatic cord exists in men. I would further train him to operate on these and on hydroceles (fluid-filled sacs that can form inside the membrane that contains the testicle).

Ambroise had been trained to treat eye problems. He would use an old-fashioned kit with all sorts of lenses and then order glasses from a bicycle-borne eyeglasses manufacturer, sponsored by Christoffel-Blindenmission, or the Christian Blind Mission (CBM). He had also been trained to do opera-tions for cataracts and has a battery-powered operating microscope and a "slit lamp" for examinations, equipment that seems to have come from the CBM. While Flore was recovering in Kijabe, Ambroise visited people around town and in nearby areas of Kenya to try to get sponsorship for more training and supplies from CBM and other organizations.

Neither Isaiah nor Ambroise are gunslingers. They do very careful, deliberate work and are cautious about the operations they take on. They will have to live with the results for a long time, as the patients will be on their doorstep forever.

The Zemio clinic has a total of fourteen employees and is supported by the fees they collect on operations, such as the $20 hernia repair they offer. AIM supplied the buildings, but they were never intended to become hospitals. They were established as midwifery clinics to help reduce the number of infant deaths at birth or soon thereafter. AIM trained midwives locally, identifying the maternal types who are the traditional birth attendants called upon during home deliveries and convincing them to bring women to the clinic because it would be cleaner than the traditional hut deliveries. The midwife's badges of honor were a little basin, a couple of sterile towels, an umbilical cord tie, and a little plastic clamp. The Azande traditionally had used cattle dung to seal umbilical cord stumps after birth, but the dung often contained a bacterium called Clostridium tetanus that causes neonatal tetanus, which killed virtually all the children who contracted the infection.

As AIM has done with the churches, I have been working to indigenize the clinics, which are now officially under the umbrella of African evangelical organizations, although that doesn't mean they are funded.

The procedures the local team had lined up for us were the types of operations we could handle given our supplies and the makeshift operating theater we had to work with. When AIM volunteer Scott Downing had joined us here in January (when we had flown down from Am Timan, Chad, carrying him with us to help with the refugees from Assa with whom he had grown up in the Congo), he had said, "This must be the world's only operating room without a single wire in the wall or outlet anywhere." I'm sure that wasn't quite accurate universally, but we were certainly far from Western medical luxury.

The Zemio clinic is a low brick building with a large room that serves as the operating theater. The windows are covered with colorful bedsheets to keep prying eyes out. The room is big enough that we can place two tables side by side, enabling us to make the most of our short time by always working on two patients at once. The recovery area is a grouping of low, wood-slatted cots. We did our consultations in a small office.

We were limited to operating during daylight hours: 6:00 a.m. to 6:00 p.m. year-round, as we are just a few degrees away from the equator. The kerosene-powered generator and battery-powered headlamps provided the only spotlights to improve visibility in the dim clinic.

We didn't have an anesthetist with us, so we could only administer local anesthetic, spinal anesthetic, or ketamine, which is a neuroleptic, not a complete anesthetic. With ketamine, the patient sometimes thrashes around, salivates excessively, and is at risk of a collapsing airway. In the United States, an anesthetist would use a sedative and an endotracheal tube. We had neither. We had atropine to help dry up patients' secretions so they wouldn't choke on their own saliva while under the influence of ketamine, but that was about it.

For these reasons, I had told the team that I did not want to do elective thyroidectomies on this trip. Doing thyroidectomies without an endotracheal tube is asking for trouble, though we have gotten away with it in the past. On our last trip to Zemio, we removed a very big goiter from a young man who thrashed around as the clamps dangled from his neck. He was not in pain—he was in a state of disoriented delirium. We had to struggle to protect the clamps and the sterile field from contamination. He wound up doing fine, but it was not a safe operation. I would be willing to do a thyroidectomy only if there were high risk of a compromised airway before we could return with an anesthetist.

Of course, the very first man we saw had a large, right-side-dominant goiter that squeezed off his airway when he turned his head. I had to admit that we needed to operate, and he was put on the next day's schedule. Later I saw a woman with a firm nodule on her thyroid gland that I thought could be follicular cancer, so she was added to the "must do" list. Another dozen patients were put on ten drops of iodine in a cup of water daily as a way of combating iodine deficiency and possibly shrinking their goiters, which was the best we could do without an injectable form of "depot" iodine, which I had successfully used in the Congo.

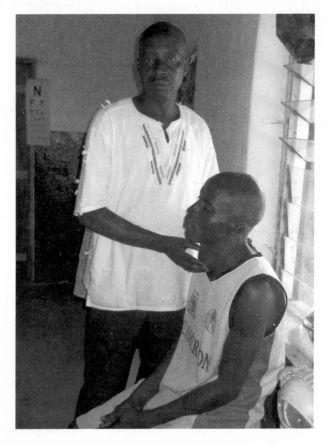

Ambroise examines a man with a large goiter. We put him on our surgical schedule.

Patients with goiters were far outnumbered by the women who arrived with downcast eyes, a hunched posture, and a shuffling gait. This evidence alone made it possible for us to diagnose at a distance, ever so astutely, pelvic inflammatory disease, or PID. The discomfort of PID is almost always secondary to the principal complaint sadly murmured by woman after woman, particularly new brides: that they had had no children. Their social value was based on this critical function, and their failure in this regard weighed heavily on them. The more frantically they pursued fertility, the more painful the act of intercourse became, a condition known as dyspareunia. And for all that pain, still no pregnancy resulted. Many said they felt that they had an abdominal mass, and some actually did. That mass was often tender and might have represented pus in the fallopian tubes or a tubo-ovarian abscess. If they weren't tender, they were likely to be benign, smooth-muscle uterine tumors called myomas; these can become very large and take over the uterus. These, of course, can cause infertility, but they sometimes also obstruct the function of other organs, like the bladder. We saw a few of these myomas, some as large as a nine-month pregnancy.

Several women asked for an operation so that they might become pregnant. Herein lies a conundrum. The operation we hope might succeed is a myomectomy; we cut the smooth-muscle tumor out of the uterine wall. If, however, the myoma occupies the whole uterus or if trying to remove it results in uncontrollable bleeding, then the uterus has to come out. I tell the patients that we will undertake an operation, but they have to sign off on it as a hysterectomy, acknowledging that sterility is one of the likely consequences—even though it is 180 degrees from their intent. And even after a successful myomectomy, the pregnancy rate is very low, since most often it is not the uterus and its lumps and bumps that were preventing pregnancy, but the plugged fallopian tubes.

We booked a half dozen hysterectomies and three or four ovarian tumor removals. All of the operative cases would require the prepackaged kits of spinal anesthetic, with which I was well supplied. During the procedure, the patients would be awake, but numb and paralyzed in the lower extremities.

Male patients often came in complaining of urinary retention, and the local practitioners and my student team almost always guessed that this was due to an enlarged prostate, or benign prostatic hypertrophy (BPH). At least a half dozen older men we saw had this complaint, but a number of them were far too young to have BPH. They often had urethral strictures or stenosis, the flip side of the same coin as PID in women—both were a consequence of the prevalence of gonorrhea.

One of the men who almost certainly did have BPH came in with quite a story. He had a distended bladder with urinary retention due to a slowly progressing urinary outlet obstruction. He had dribbled with overflow incontinence for a while but then had prolonged periods of total urinary obstruction. If his problem is a complete obstruction of the urethra, a catheter cannot be passed to relieve him. But, at the same time, it isn't possible to go for weeks, months, or years without passing urine!

"So how is it that he relieves himself of the urinary backup?" I asked.

Ambroise spoke to the man in Pazande. The man withdrew from the folds of his clothing an old syringe and held it out silently.

"Does he undergo bladder puncture with that?"

"Yes," Ambroise told me.

"How often?"

"Two to three times each day."

Two to three times each day with a syringe he carries in his pocket!

The man needed a prostatectomy. I knew I could do it, but as I'd learned in Malawi and elsewhere, it's vital to the operation that the nursing staff clearly understands how to keep the urinary catheter clear of clots. The operation and recovery typically requires a three-way catheter, which does not exist here. Instead, we would have to insert a Foley catheter below through the urethra and insert another one above, into the bladder, as a suprapubic catheter—a catheter inserted directly into the bladder through the abdominal wall—to use in through-and-through irrigation, pumping in saline that will then flow out of the urethral catheter. The nursing staff must irrigate these catheters to prevent clots. If there is a clot, the situation quickly becomes an emergency.

I agreed to do the prostatectomy if the nurses were drilled for at least a day on how to care for a catheter and how to use suprapubic flow-through to clear clots. In the past, I'd worked with nurses who were resistant to dealing with these catheters. In one case, the local surgeon in Chad insisted that a suprapubic catheter was the cause of all infections and proved his authority by going around and pulling out the suprapubic catheters immediately after the operation, despite orders to the contrary. The patients had to return to the OR for another spinal anesthetic and a repeat operation—not once, but twice! I'd seen other similar cases of incorrect catheter care in other environments, and in one, a man died as a result of the bladder blowout that followed the formation of clots. I had trained the staff that performed this operation, so I felt a sense of responsibility, despite the fact that I wasn't there at the time.

So, I insisted that these nurses be fully prepared.

Another man was seen for a mass in his scrotum. It was adjacent to the testis, tender, and did not transluminate—a fancy word for whether light from, say, a flashlight shines through it or not. Hydroceles (accumulations of fluid in the internal membranes of the scrotum), for example, do transluminate. I determined that this man had a varicocele—a dilation in the testicular veins that run along the spermatic artery. These veins return the blood from the scrotum to inside the body, creating a countercurrent heat-exchange system that keeps the testes cooler than the body, creating the right environment for sperm to form.

The varicocele was an innocent abnormality, except that it would raise the temperature of the testes' blood supply to that of the body. The pooling of the warmer blood in the varicocele would lead to infertility—one reason to surgically correct the problem.

So we asked this fellow how many children he had, expecting none or very few. The Pazande speakers burst out in laughter when he replied, "Twenty-three."

Yeah, right! They repeated the question in French.

"*Vingt-trois,*" he said. We told him that was unlikely.

"Twenty-three!" he repeated.

Okay, okay, we said. Well, the varicocele was of no consequence, since he had proven his virility—his net worth—already. We told him he could be on his way, that no operation was necessary.

I turned to the team after he had gone. "Maternity is a matter of fact," I said. "Paternity a matter of opinion."

What to say about hernias? We saw patients with almost every kind known in the medical books—abdominal, femoral, and inguinal; direct and indirect; acquired and congenital. I gave a short dissertation in response to a question from Joe: "Why are there so many hernias around here?" It is the difference between a prevalence and an incidence, a stock and a flow. The number of hernias in a population like this is high because whatever was here is still here, since no one else has been fixing them. This means we are seeing the natural history of the disease without intervention. The congenital hernias would happen anywhere, but elsewhere they would be found and fixed. Not here. Direct hernias are more frequently acquired than congenital, and there is good cause. This population is quite familiar with lifting, with straining to pass urine, with chronic coughs (such as with tuberculosis), with increased intra-abdominal pressure due to constipation from dehydration.

We saw several hernias that needed fixing and would benefit from a mesh implant. The Zemio clinic, of course, had none, but fortunately we had packed a good sheet and many smaller ones, enough to stock the station for years. The mesh implant is a simple product that is ridiculously expensive, a twenty-cent piece of material that carries multiple millions in liability risk. The mesh typically costs more than all of the operations we would be doing that week. A little piece is typically charged as the whole sheet, but we were using the extra mesh from the oversize sheets (which would've been discarded in the first world) to make many smaller, single-use patches. Our patients would get expensive mesh without the costs that are usually carried along with it.

One of the women with a self-diagnosed abdominal mass had come for an operation. I discovered quickly that her mass was actually ascites, an accumulation of fluid in the abdomen, caused by portal hypertension, probably a result of cirrhosis of the liver. Portal hypertension results from restricted blood flow from the gastrointestinal tract to the liver. Fluid is transuded (passed through, like perspiration) from the higher pressures in the portal system and retained in the peritoneal cavity. We told her she did *not* need an operation and instead needed a medicine we had right here—furosemide, a diuretic. An hour later, I saw the woman stop Mary Anne Harris, who was walking up the path from the church to the main house. She talked with Mary Anne in a mendicant posture—hands outstretched in a cupped position and knees bent in a curtsy.

Mary Anne asked me about her later, saying that the assigned operation fees Ambroise set were more than she could pay. Curious and confused—we hadn't even recommended an operation—I asked how much it was. Ambroise tries to keep the staff and the operations going here year-round based on the operations and care we give in a week. As all of our services and equipment and drugs are donated, this is the only time of the year when their "payday" comes through. I want to know little about and interfere less with this system. I am convinced that free services are worthless, and that for care to be sustainable, the patient has to have skin in the game. Patients need to value the service to the degree of partial participation or the therapy won't be effective; they can see the enormous resource expenditure on their behalf, and some part of this should support the ongoing services in the clinic. Mary Anne told me she heard that the operation cost 20,000 Central African francs, or about US $40.

For a major operation and hospitalization—if we might glorify the minimal bed and family care offered at Zemio clinic as such—and all the drugs and sutures and disposables involved, this is a real bargain, but it is also very expensive given that the salary for a full day's work is $1 for most laborers in the CAR, $2 for a skilled workman. That means that the least of our operations is equivalent to a month's work. That is okay with me as long as it keeps the clinic in operation and there is no skimming of the proceeds.

But this was all beside the point. "This is the woman with ascites," I told Mary Anne, "and she either misunderstood all that we just told her about her treatment—because she is not getting an operation—or something else is going on." After a further explanation, the woman was still asking for help from Mary Anne. There were three possible explanations. First, the people here may not feel they have any other way of attracting outside support except by displaying their disabilities and illnesses. I don't want the traveling team or the local workers to be abused. We cannot be so successful in our generosity that we are drained to the point of going out of business, a concern I was feeling acutely on this expedition. The second possibility is that the Zande patients, having seen me here before, dismiss medicine as second-class treatment. The only *real* therapy comes from a direct and immediate surgical cure, they think, so they seek out an operation even when advised that they don't need it.

A third explanation was made clear to me much later. Isaiah presented me with an extensive logbook of operations and the "charges" for these services, which few, if any, of the patients could pay. They were maintaining the logbook to impress upon the patients the fees for these services. But to my surprise, Isaiah turned the charges over to me to pay; it was what I owed for operating for free and for donating supplies! At the end of it all, in addition to my transportation expenses and room and board, the patient charges totaled several thousand dollars. In essence, I was paying patients to undergo operations I provided to them for free. I was even presented with costs for patients whom we referred to Ambroise or Isaiah, to be seen after I left. Isaiah shrugged and smiled, passing me the logbook with a question that was quite reasonable in his mind: "From where else could we ever get such support for these expensive services?"

On our first evening, during our after-dinner tutorial, as drowsy as we were with jet lag and the tropical heat and humidity that precede the nocturnal rainstorms during this season, the team was still on a bit of a buzz. "I can't believe I'm really here" was passing into "Now just what am I going to do with this once-in-a-lifetime opportunity?" It was the first time some had ever been off their home continent. It was the first time one had ever been in a medical setting. For one, it was the first time he had ever been in an operating room, and for others, it was the first opportunity to learn and perform procedures.

The team had been discovering itself and now believed what I had been telling them: This was the surgical team with perhaps the greatest potential we had fielded, and we could expect to do great things in teaching the indigenous staff and moving them up to a considerably higher level of capability.

With those thoughts in their minds, they went to bed anticipating the first operating day of the expedition.

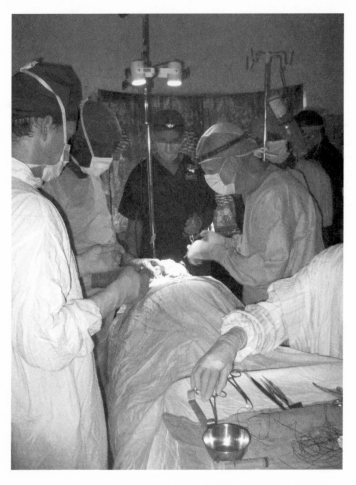

One of our first thyroidectomies in Zemio, expertly handled by Ambroise with support from the local and visiting teams.

CHAPTER FOUR

DAY ONE IN THE THEATER

June 5–6, 2012, Zemio mission station

THE MORNING OF OUR OPENING DAY IN THE ZEMIO MISSION station offered us the rare treat of a good, relaxed breakfast; we usually make rounds on the post-op patients first, but as yet we had none. The night was entertaining, though possibly not very restful, for those team members who had never enjoyed the rainy season in a tropical forest under a pan roof. The stately avenue of mango trees dropped heavily sodden fruit onto the metal roofs as the rain poured down. The rains came late this year, so the mangoes were in peak fruiting—much to the delight of the fruit bats, which were squeaking and squabbling all night long. With a foot-wide wingspan that enables them to carry off a ripe mango, they forage by night and carry the spoils back to their roost—unless they bomb our roofs with it while we try to sleep. It was not that long ago, a couple of decades maybe, that the elephants would come right through the station and vacuum up the mangoes and distribute their pips far and wide, planting them all along the river with their ready-made fertilizer.

This area is a game refuge, so designated by the CAR to accord with the Azande's hunter-gatherer lifestyle. But there are more people here now than there were twenty years ago, with the influx of DRC refugees and the arrival of the Mbororo cattle herders (a subgroup of the Fulani ethnic group), who have increasingly moved south and eastward from the west African Sahel to graze their cattle in the protected savannah and forest. This cattle driving isn't authorized, but there is hardly a real central government presence here to repel them. And that is also the chief reason that the Lord's Resistance Army (LRA) and the Uganda People's Defence Force (UPDF) have migrated into this area; it is a refuge from which they can strike freely into neighboring countries. This region of the CAR may have the boundaries of a sovereign nation-state, but it is powerless to defend and protect itself. Neither of these outside armies would be here if there were a real entity to block them.

Despite the overgrowth of the human population in the area, marauding wildlife is still a concern for the local agronomists. Herds of bongo or other antelope come into their gardens and enjoy the feast offered by the land. Red colobus monkeys come in hordes and pull out everything edible. And still the most effective destroyer of the tribe's *shambas* ("gardens" in Kiswahili) is a band of elephants, which can clear a whole village's annual production in a matter of an hour on any given night. The villagers post sentries with sticks and bang on drums, but those are hardly disincentives to a hungry elephant.

One of our patients the previous day had reminded us of the dominance of wildlife in the area, particularly in previous decades. A Bantu man sat in the chair, pulled off his shirt, and explained that he had a bothersome condition he wished to have fixed with an operation. He had a small jagged scar on his lower-right chest, below his right nipple. In his back, just to the right of his spine, he had a much larger scar. It was retracted and had a small sinus tract in the base. He complained that when he lay down at night, fluid would drain from the scar on his back. That was it—no fever, no weight loss, no signs of chronic illness or pain. Yet this had been going on for some time. When we asked how long, we were told twenty-two years. How did this come about?

In 1990, the man explained, he had a run-in with a bull elephant. The elephant charged and gored him, pushing a tusk into and through him and pinning him into the swampy marsh. The animal then pulled his tusk out and left the man stuck there, where he was later found and brought into the village for help. I could hardly believe the story, given that he was sitting in front of me, alive and well twenty-two years later, complaining only of a minor sinus tract fistula from what was probably osteomyelitis, or an infected bone, as a result of a still-present foreign body!

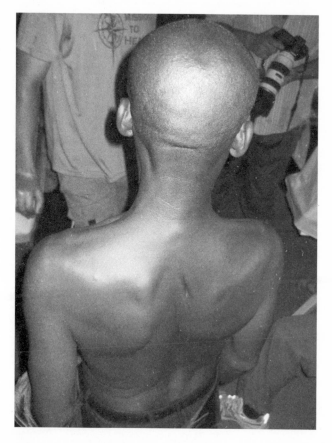

A man who was gored through and through by an elephant and survived with only a weeping scar.

That morning, though, there were no elephants meandering along the tree-lined boulevards of the Zemio mission station. We did hear fruit bats rustling and dropping mangoes. We also spotted monkeys as well as a lone civet cat rustling though the leaves. There is also abundant bird life, whose familiar chorus serves as a dawn wake-up call. The raucous guinea fowl acts as a security system, setting off a howling response to the animal intruders who come to raid the gardens.

Our examination of the wildlife had to come to a quick end, though, given the operations we had ahead of us: an ovarian cyst, five big hernias, a large goiter, and a hysterectomy for a much-enlarged uterus with a giant myoma. And the consultations would continue in between.

In the clinic, I did consultations with Ambroise and at least one medical student while periodically calling on the adjacent operating theater to prep patients on the simple wooden platforms that served as operating tables. We always try to fill both operating tables, although our rhythm isn't always perfect on opening day. The morning consultations were a string of "same same but different" patients—a phrase I borrowed from a shop sign in the Ladakh region of India, and which many of my patients in Africa use to describe their condition. Each comes in with much the same problem as his or her neighbors, but there's always a twist based on the individual's circumstances; thus the "same" is "different." Some of these conditions are tragic and some treatable, but they are all representative of the struggles of the African "burden of disease" and the counter-matching efforts we must make in doing this work.

Repairing hernias highlights one of our greatest challenges: discovering and treating the underlying causes of a malady. An elderly woman came in with two lateral lumbar triangle hernias. I asked when she had first noted them. In the past few months, she told me. They presented a great opportunity from a teaching perspective: Because there were two, it would be possible to do one myself and instruct someone through the other.

"Why might I ask her about the onset of the hernias?" I asked the students. "These are two relatively easy hernias to fix."

They got it right: Because we learned that she had just recently acquired them, there was quite possibly a specific reason for them. It would be best for us to discover the primary cause; if we didn't address it, any repair would be likely to fail. The typical reason for the appearance of an acquired hernia is increased pressure in the abdomen because of an enlarged prostate, a bowel obstruction, or a chronic cough. Any of these problems would cause an immediate recurrence of the hernia if it isn't addressed. If they are ruled out and the hernia is simply the result of injury or of the attenuated abdominal wall giving way, we might anticipate a successful repair. But we have to investigate first. Like all things here, however, that is easier said than done. Diagnostic equipment is limited.

In this woman, we could feel the hernias easily, but as I began to explore her abdomen, I found a lax abdominal wall, and through it, I could clearly feel a very large, moveable, and solid mass that seemed to hang down from and be connected to the liver. It was not an enlarged uterus or any mass associated with the pelvic organs, or I might have suspected a potential ovarian tumor. When I continued my exam and found that the whites of her eyes were slightly yellowed, the diagnosis became abundantly and unfortunately clear. She had a large, late-stage hepatoma, or liver cancer.

We explained that she did not need an operation. In the United States, she might have received an enthusiastic program of operation, radiation, and chemotherapy, but even then, the effort would have been to little purpose. The life expectancy even with operation is very rarely greater than six months. And here, if we were to attempt a surgical intervention, she would have to leave the village and spend the rest of her life in an ICU, strapped down and separated from all supportive family. Her life expectancy would be the same, but she would be as ostracized as those local criminals who are exiled to the "Village of Murderers." And the cost to attempt to prolong the life of this one individual? The entire GDP of this region.

For this woman and for the whole of the Zemio subprefecture, such options are unknown and wouldn't have been available anyway. Were she treated, a hospital would squander scores of units of blood for transfusions and monopolize sophisticated operating rooms and radiotherapy devices to no avail. So in a way, her lack of access to treatment was fortunate: Application of any or all of these intensive care services for a problem at that stage is futile and carries with it the tragedy of isolation from family at a time when she needs them most.

I explained the situation to an accompanying family member and gave her ten pills. "When it hurts a lot, take two; and when the pain is unbearable, take the remaining eight." This is called "compression of morbidity and maximization of residual life."

I always make a distinction between resectability and operability. Resectability refers to the tumor; it is a judgment on whether the tumor can be removed completely and successfully. Operability, on the other hand, is not a function of the tumor; it's a function of the patient. It is possible to have a resectable tumor in an inoperable patient, such as someone with chronic lung disease with a small tumor in the already-diseased lung. Yet neither resectability nor operability determines whether an operation *should* be done. That is a matter of greater judgment. With Flore, I had made the judgment in one direction, but in this case it did not make any sense to operate.

Of course, the people with me don't always agree with my judgments. Dan Vryhof hadn't agreed that bringing Flore out of the CAR was the right choice at the time. Before that, on a mission in the Himalayas, I had with me a jeweler from Chicago who was acting as our translator. Our first patient, a grandmother, had a hepatoma like our current patient. It involved each of the liver lobes. Even if it had been resectable, the woman was inoperable. She had such little protein in her diet that she wouldn't be able to tolerate an incision, let alone a big operation. And we had none of the supplies or resources to make it possible anyway. As I was explaining this to her daughter and giving her the pills for compression of morbidity, the translator—who spoke Hindi while these people spoke Ladakhi, so we were playing telephone, with three-step translation—stopped abruptly and said, "You can't say that!"

"This means she'll be with her family until her life is unbearable," I explained.

"No!" the translator replied. "We've got to get a helicopter here and bring her to Delhi to have an operation." I tried to explain the lack of wisdom in what she was saying, that she was talking about investing massive resources to prolong this old woman's life by about a month, but she wouldn't hear it. She halted the ongoing operations of the clinic and our consultations with other patients and ran around trying to get people to sponsor this grandmother for evacuation for futile advanced care. Eventually, I stopped her and told her it was time for her to go back to Delhi so that the rest of us could get on with taking care of treatable patients. If any one of the imported team members diverts more than 10 percent of my attention away from the patients, he or she has to go.

If Flore's situation had been different, if she had been elderly or childless, or if there had been other limiting factors, we wouldn't have made the choices we did.

It was a very big opening day, including quite a few firsts. Under my assistance, Bruce and Claudia did their first-ever spinal anesthetic lumbar punctures. It was Joe's first time ever in an operating room. Josh started his first IV and also scrubbed in for the first time. And I helped Isaiah do his first femoral hernia, which requires sewing with a big needle right over the exposed femoral vein— big, blue, and terribly daunting. Older literature refers to it as "the vein of death."

Between operations, we saw more patients and added more operations to our list. One man had a very large, soft, benign tumor (a lipoma) in his thigh. It looked like a big case I could turn over to Josh and Dan, who were eager to see as many lumps and bumps as possible—and this was a big one for a student case.

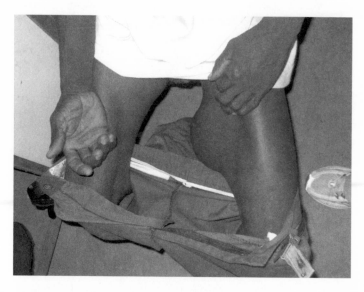

A large benign tumor, or lipoma, on the patient's thigh that would make a perfect teaching case.

Possibly the most astounding consult of the day, though, was with a man with a huge hydrocele and elephantiasis of the scrotum. Like that of the man who claimed he had fathered twenty-three children the day before, the diagnosis was fairly quick, particularly because this man's hydrocele was the size of a soccer ball! It was two and a half liters in capacity, about ten pounds, and looked even larger on his thin frame. He had calluses on the bottom of his scrotum from dragging it and sitting on it. We put him on the schedule for the next day. We would be doing the entire operation under superficial lidocaine injection! It was the best option available to us.

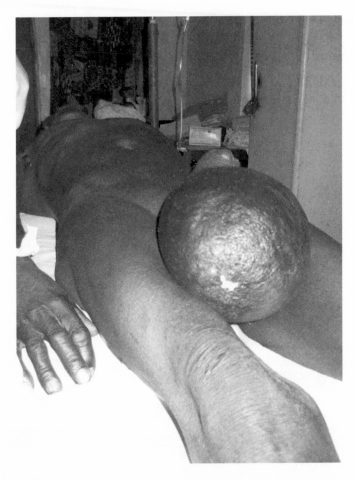

A poor fellow with a 2½ liter hydrocele resulting from Wuchereria bancrofti filariasis infection.

Again, we had to discuss the underlying cause, which was the same for this man as for the woman who followed him. She had elephantiasis of the lower extremities. Her legs were hugely swollen with lymph, the left much larger than the right. The cause? An infected and obstructed lymphatic drainage system. And the cause of that? Wuchereria bancrofti, a parasitic filaria (nematode worm), one of the cardinal "neglected tropical diseases." The filarial parasite itself is the carrier of another bacterium called Wolbachia. We treated the filariasis with an agent called ivermectin but also gave tetracycline for the filarial parasite's own infection of Wolbachia. The bacterium is probably responsible for the lymphangitis (inflammation of the lymph vessels) that results in lymphatic scarring and elephantiasis.

Another of our hernia patients had an enlarged left lower leg, with the kinds of granular inflammations I have seen only in podoconiosis, or mossy foot. This is a disabling elephantiasis that results from an inflammation of the lymph system caused by some of the clay silica and iron contents of the soils in this part of the world. In this area, filarial infection is a more common cause of elephantiasis, but each form is found here: one caused by a mosquito-borne parasite, the other by the constituents of the very ground we walk on—in their case, barefoot.

These cases as well as more consults at the OR door, appearing for help with patients with hernias, uterine myomas, and ovarian cysts, prompted me to repeat the fact that the natural progression of these conditions was visible here, whereas the overly abundant and redundant health-care systems in other first-world countries would have treated them long before they had progressed to the point that we were seeing. Would filarial infestation result in severe lymphedema or elephantiasis if it occurred in the United States? Not likely.

Flore's disease had reached a point that it wouldn't have in the United States, too, although her tumor grew so fast that it's hard to be sure. Once she was at

Kijabe, we learned why it had done so, a reason I had suspected but had no way to verify. She was HIV seropositive.

When I heard the news from Ambroise, I immediately responded that he should work to get her started on highly active antiretroviral therapy (HAART). It turned out that in Obo, there was a group that had acquired free HAART drugs from the World Health Organization. While some might wonder whether Flore's HIV status made our decision a poor one, we didn't view it that way. In some ways, she became an index patient. Her family members and others in the community have begun to get tested, and as more people are found to be positive, they too are seeking treatment.

At the pole of inaccessibility, the population has been relatively out of reach of everything, including AIDS. HIV infection has not yet become a rampant problem. Many of the people who live here aren't aware of it and certainly don't recognize the signs and symptoms as the disease progresses to the frank findings of late-stage AIDS. Flore's husband, we eventually realized, was a classic case. The problem is that AIDS follows armies and commerce, and as the LRA moved into the area, with its propensity for rape, and was followed by the African Union forces, primarily the UPDF, they brought HIV from more populated—and "accessible"—areas with them. Sadly, with a couple of $20 bills in their pockets, the members of these armies have more wealth than many of the people here can imagine, and that earns them certain privileges, such as never sleeping alone. A passing army opens up the brothels of big-city slums to the pole of inaccessibility. Thus, AIDS follows roads.

Yet now, through Flore, certain benefits such as HIV testing and HAART drugs, which are now available for free, are becoming accessible to the people in Obo. Through our intervention with Flore, we have floated all boats in Obo, and, we hope, have saved untold lives simply by spreading awareness.

The operations throughout the day were, for the most part, done well and with much help from the indigenous staff, exactly as they should be. Of course, nothing is ever quite that simple, so we did have one major complication—the one I predicted. We got away with the ketamine use in the young man with the large goiter. I helped Ambroise do the thyroidectomy. But in the afternoon, we had a traumatic experience with a woman undergoing a hysterectomy. We were removing her enlarged, fibroid-filled uterus, but the spinal anesthetic administered was not completely successful and was supplemented by a ketamine injection. Then she needed more ketamine, and she got more.

Then, it happened. She began shrieking and wailing in a mournful cry and thrashing about, not from pain but from hallucinations. She was having a ketamine-induced psychotic break. Adults, particularly in the indigenous people we treat, are more likely to hallucinate when stimulated by ketamine. Unlike children, who are more likely to experience free-floating anxiety on ketamine, adults have a wealth of real-life threats to hallucinate about and plenty of disturbing situations to flash back to. Frankly, having your belly open is stimulation enough. The risk of hallucinations like this is why I was so opposed to using the ketamine as our principle anesthetic agent for adults.

We were almost finished, but she was straining and pushing out her gut. We had no hope of closing the incision. We couldn't achieve hemostasis— the securing of bleeding small vessels—so we could suture the clamped veins and arteries in the broad ligament, which connects the uterus to the walls and floor of the pelvis. We needed to give her an injection of an antipsychotic agent, like diazepam (Valium) or phenothiazine (Thorazine), or any narcotic or muscle relaxant. But we had none of the above. We had to hold her down as she wailed. Suddenly, her O$_2$ saturation began to drop (thank God for the pulse oximeter!). We began rubbing her clavicles to stimulate her.

As in all things urgent, Claudia went back and rummaged through our supplies again. Miraculously, in our stock of miscellaneous drugs she found a single ampoule of diazepam. With the first hit of Valium, the patient immediately became peaceful, and the abdominal wall relaxed, allowing us to finish the procedure and get her safely closed.

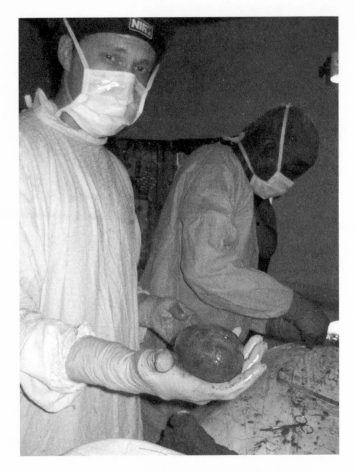

Dan holding the goiter of a man who, after receiving ketamine,
sang hymns in French and Pazande.

You never know what response you'll get from ketamine, which makes it dangerous. It has achieved popularity in much of the developing world because it can be given by a nonanesthetist—the patient's blood pressure or pulse is usually not adversely affected. It is not my anesthetic of choice, although it can be useful, and I wouldn't necessarily pass up the kind of response we got from the young man with the goiter. As we completed his thyroidectomy, he peacefully serenaded us with hymns of praise in French and Pazande. The stark contrast in their responses made me consider the possibility that these two patients had led very different lives.

At the evening tutorial, it was hard to hold the team down. It was a good group and they were all working together in common purpose without a lot of interjected ego. Each reported on what he or she had seen and done, many for the first time and despite the fact that some are adjuncts in the health-care field.

We spent some time discussing the beliefs of the people here. Animism is dominant, and the stories that surround the "spirits" and the havoc they wreak when disturbed are rampant. Despite the growth of various forms of Christianity in the region, belief in witchcraft is still common. In our line of work, we would hear a lot about "causative agents"—particularly curses that result when somebody disturbs the spirit of that tree or this rock or the water witch who lives in the river. The people here believe that unless you find the person who cast the curse, whether accidentally or with purpose, and affix blame, the curse will not be ended.

There is a pastor whose grave is prominent on the mission station between the church and the main house. He had gone to the United States for two years, and when he returned, his son came across the Mbomou River from the DRC in a dugout canoe loaded with buffalo meat for a celebration. But the canoe swamped, and the pastor's son was swept away and never recovered. There are quite a few crocodiles in parts of the river.

The Azande insisted that the only thing that would bring closure to the pastor after this tragic loss was for him to identify and denounce the culprit who had wished this curse upon him. He said no, that this was an accident, and there was no one at fault. But there are no accidents in Zande land. The pastor was pressed further to identify and denounce the culprit. He refused. He was incarcerated and kept there until he would confess. If he was going to protect the identity of this malefactor he would be, in American legalese, "an unindicted coconspirator." Pushed further to bear witness to the miscreant, he was steadfast and was consequently so devalued in status among the Azande that he was essentially ostracized from that time until his death.

If something negative happens, it has to be someone's fault. Although it's becoming more and more rare, the Azande still use diviners to determine culpability. Once a culprit has been identified, the proof is uncovered by a Zande diviner through the "poison oracle," benge, which has a strychnine base. The diviner prepares the poison and then sits with the accuser (who is sometimes the same person as the diviner) and the accused, as well as a few witnesses, chanting until the spirits move the diviner to some kind of clairvoyance. The diviner makes an incantation: "Oh benge, benge, if this man is sleeping with this other man's wife, kill this chicken!" A small pullet is seized and dosed with the benge. The diviner asks the question at hand in a variety of ways to clarify the message to the oracle, sometimes asking the oracle to kill the chicken and sometimes asking the oracle to save it. If the pullet falls over dead, the ceremony might be repeated—it could have been a false positive. If the suspect's guilt is confirmed, the offended can then legitimately impose a curse. And if someone is known to have been cursed, that curse is usually fulfilled—somehow.

This process might be replaced or followed by the ritual of the judgment tree, under which the paramount chief hears and judges cases. Chief Sasa, of the Assa group of the Azande, ruled by hereditary right, and he had legal authority to impose capital punishment. He was said to be a benevolent fellow since he killed no one. He instead would judge the evidence and if the convicted were found guilty, he would send them into internal exile in the Village of Murderers. A person so ostracized could not contact any of his or her family or other tribal clansmen and was left to his or her own solitary devices, utterly isolated. And yet, Chief Sasa might as well have issued a death sentence: In the Village of Murderers, life expectancy was measured in weeks. They simply died. As social animals dependent on their community, they could not continue.

The Azande are mainly afraid of the water and do not spend time fishing in the big waters of their river. And they certainly would not go swimming for entertainment. If they do go fishing, it is usually with a spear, and they stalk through the muddy shallows of the marsh spearing the catfish that wriggle down into the mud, trying to make enough of a cocoon to survive through the dry season; when the rains come and flood the pan again, the catfish wriggle out of their encasement and swim off. But if Azande go near the river, they do so timorously, convinced that there are water sprites and evil spirits abounding in that treacherous area. They can all cite quite a few examples of people who were so possessed that they took off into the bush at the river's edge, dived into the waters, and were not heard from again.

We have our own totems in the West, ranging from black cats to broken mirrors to spilled salt to two-headed anythings. The "primitives" who carry on superstitions and rituals like the Azande's are not apart from us. And we all have rituals to protect ourselves.

One complicated ritual we face is the disposal of resected body parts. I have been asked when removing body parts, such as goiters, to carry the specimen to the family. They might choose to carry it out into the forest and bury it. In the West, we face the same type of disposal problem—for example, at what stage do the "products of conception" go to the lab for examination and incineration rather than to the morgue for a funeral?

As I wrote these thoughts in my journal in the dark by headlamp, insects swarming around the LED screen and the light on my forehead, I decided that the "scientific" disposal I follow in these places is much the same as a traditional Western burial—a ritual of respect for what is or had been, at least in part, human, and deserving of greater respect than composting.

As would become our usual ritual, I organized the group for a five o'clock wake-up on the second day of operations, and at six o'clock we walked over to the "hospital," where we made rounds on the post-op patients. They were all doing well, including those whose operations had been done under minimal local anesthesia. Five men who'd had hernia operations were sitting with their hands raised over their heads in the usual group salute: "*Sene foro!*" They expressed their gratitude with smiles and thank-yous. "*Merci mengi!*"

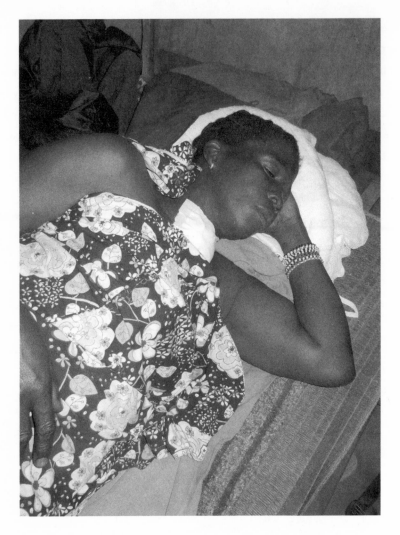

One of our thyroidectomy patients successfully recovering post-op.

We returned to have breakfast before we began our seven o'clock duties at the theater. And in a light sprinkle of rain, Josh and I walked toward the theater from breakfast dressed in our OR scrubs. As we did so we saw a fellow pursuing us on his *velo* (bicycle) who seemed intent on seeing me before we went in. After the usual greetings, in his case a bit more exuberant and persistent than most, he started to tell me something about a thyroidectomy. I thought he might be related to the fellow on whom we had done the thyroidectomy yesterday, the patient who had sung hymns in Pazande and French. I nodded, agreeing that the patient was doing well. He pointed to me and I agreed that I was doing fine as well, thank you. He persisted, pointing to himself and then to me and sweeping with a hand over the river below the bluff.

Then it dawned on me. When he referred to himself, he pointed to his neck. There was a very fine, thin line and a well-healed incision—a reminder of our prior encounter. I had told Josh in our tutorial the night before that it was likely a patient would not remember the doctor who had once given him a prescription that may have cured him; however, if he has a scar, it is a memorial of the event (good or otherwise), and the patient is likely to remember the time a surgeon separated him from a disease. And here he was. He had come from the other side of the refugee settlement when he heard I was here again. He had not been here when I was visiting three months ago, but vowed he would come on his bicycle to visit when I returned.

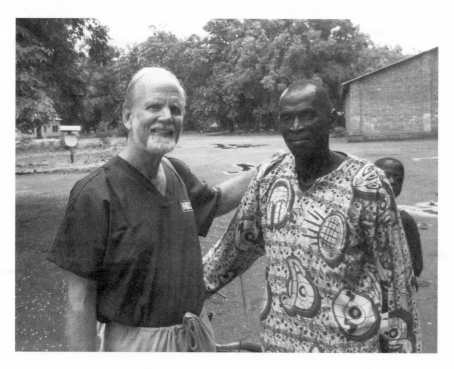

A man who came to thank me for a thyroidectomy I had done on him twenty-four years before.

I had operated on him twenty-four years before in Assa. I might not have remembered his name or identity, but he certainly would remember this white man, no matter how strange his name or how far he traveled to come here. He wanted to express again his gratitude as he pointed to my "signature" in his neck. He had a strong voice and normal thyroid function, as far as I could tell. Given the excessive length of his incision, his goiter likely exceeded a kilogram in size. And here he was, pumping his bicycle uphill to make a post-op courtesy call, a quarter century from an event many in the Western world would have eventually forgotten.

We always have a stutter start to the day, and there is a lag between arrival at the work site and any work getting done, since first there are inquiries as to how the night has gone and what the health of all family members might be. Once these conversations are complete, everybody knows that the "doctor is in" and the queue of consults at the OR door begins, continuing as long as the "market is open." We fall back into our routine, setting up in the scrub chamber adjacent to the theater and conducting consultations as we wait for the OR to be ready. We have a number of operations to get to in a given day, so the rush is on.

Our operative lists and interval consultations at the OR antechamber continue. The team circles around to view the incoming patients and their pathology while also working with the local staff to shuttle the instruments out to the "autoclave"—the pressure cookers over the kerosene stove we purchased in Uganda as well as a bigger pressure cooker over a wood fire, blackened by the smoke, that gives us our next case's recycled instruments, gowns, and drapes. We packed in gowns and gloves, and after use they are washed before going into our pressure-cooker autoclave—even the allegedly "disposable" paper ones—and hung out on the bushes to dry and get the UV "sterilization" of the equatorial sunshine. Sometimes, we have to put them on wet, and sometimes they are still hot from the pot.

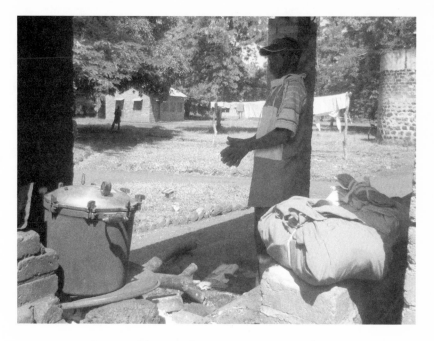

Our state-of-the-art sterilizing system—a pressure cooker over
a wood fire—with stacks of linens waiting to be cleaned.

All of this "stuff" originated in the mission control room in the Derwood basement, making its way from first-world redundancy to a place where the needs far outstrip the supplies. Whatever is considered disposable in the developed world is here reused until it literally falls apart. But the shortage is in both equipment and skill. We can jettison the equipment with ease and without obligation. The skill with which it is to be used comes at a higher cost in personal commitment—from both sides.

This is why each day must present teaching opportunities. It is still a surprise to me that each of the CFAs, though they have been in the OR often and have seen many procedures done, have never actually performed spinal anesthetics and other basic procedures. For example, as long as Leenta had been assisting in operations, she'd been holding retractors for someone else while they suture; she had never done any suturing herself. Not only did she place her first sutures and do her first ties, she also did them on the very same patient on whom she'd done the preparation and the spinal. And she did so with no more than a little help because the instruction we gave to the patient to bend forward had not resulted in any other posture than a straight back, even though we reinforced it with examples. Nevertheless, Leenta got it done. She then assisted in the operation, including the deep ties, an item of great consequence to the patient's well-being. She then closed the skin. And about time, too! Highly possessive and liability-shy doctors had not allowed her any of these three opportunities. Here, she said she got all three in the same patient; already a worthwhile reason for repeating the mission—quite apart from its nonmedical and nonsurgical rewards—whatever its expenses in cost and inconveniences!

We did the drill—preparation, positioning, projection, and penetration—with each person who would perform a spinal anesthetic so that he or she would be ready to feel the "pop" as the slender needle is pushed through the meninges. We discussed the importance of limiting the anesthetic and mixing it with enough glucose, which is heavy, to ensure that it stays inside the dura to affect only the lower nerves and numb only the abdomen and lower extremities. If it is injected too rapidly, it could make for turbulence, and the turmoil of the flow would cause it to rise higher than we wish. If the patient immediately lies down, the anesthetic agent, depending on how much sugar is in it, could roll to the bottom of the dural sheath within the spinal canal and move up too high. If it goes up to cervical spine levels and numbs the origins of the phrenic nerve, the patient does not breathe—this is called a "high spinal." And we don't have the equipment or ability to insert endotracheal tubes. We monitor the blood pressure and keep an IV open to infuse fluid, since the "capacitance reservoirs" are also paralyzed and the loss of this vascular tone would result in pooling of blood. So we need the patient monitored with an IV, a pulse oximeter, and a blood pressure cuff or a Propaq monitor. We also have a Foley catheter in the bladder, since there is no ability to sense bladder fullness; if it is a long case, or if a lot of fluid is infused, the urinary retention and bladder distension can make it impossible for the patient to pee after the spinal anesthetic has worn off. So, the four Ps—preparation, positioning, projection, and penetration—especially a swift and efficient penetration, makes everything look easy. Yet there is very little forgiveness in the fragile, sterile environment of the central nervous system.

As we did the consultations, I assisted Ambroise or Isaiah as necessary. Isaiah was doing a very good job on indirect inguinal hernias but had a rather proscribed boundary around what he could and could not do. He had never done a femoral hernia before yesterday, so I said I would help him do the one we had scheduled today, and a second one was performed with even less of my help. With my assistance he did it as well as I might have with him assisting me. And it was a pleasure to strip off the gloves and let Emmanuel take over as first assistant to help Isaiah complete it. The very big hydrocele represented another class of patients Isaiah was not authorized to attempt to repair, but it is an easily teachable operation. I took him through the procedure—an inversion of the hydrocele lining that I call a "water bottle" repair—notably without Ambroise scrubbing. In this procedure, a linear incision is made in the distended sac and a geyser of fluid is drained away. Then, the sac is inverted to close the secreting lining inside out. With the cavity thus obliterated, no more fluid can accumulate.

Joe had been taking photos and felt more comfortable looking through the lens, saying that this was the first time he had seen the human intestine. He was taking notes outside the operating room and asking some questions, such as the difference between sharp (cutting) dissection and blunt (tearing) dissection. Making an interesting assumption, Joe asked, "How many other doctors are there here in Zemio?"

"Zero," I replied. "The only doctor here is the one going back on the plane with you." Not everyone who can operate or is being taught to do so is a doctor.

"I wouldn't give a fig for the simplicity on this side of complexity," said Oliver Wendell Holmes, "but I would give my right arm for the simplicity on the far side of complexity." Our goal on this trip is to get to that far-side simplicity—the simplicity of necessity.

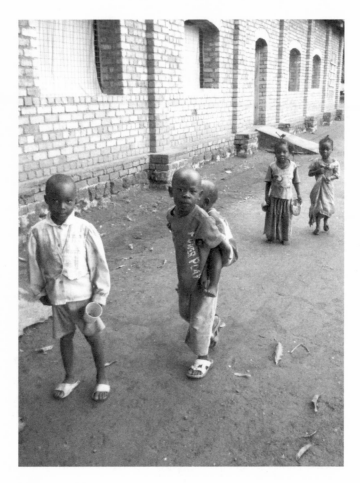

Five little ones, one of the older siblings carrying the youngest on his back, traveling by the clinic.

CHAPTER FIVE

BY COAT HANGER
OR PICKUP OR CELL PHONE

June 7, 2012, Zemio mission station

WE HAD OUR OWN ENCOUNTER WITH A TOTEM ON THE MORNING OF our third day in Zemio, or at least Bruce did. If there was a snake-phobe among us, it was Bruce, the Muskegon hunter. In fact, he had bad dreams of a snake crawling through the window and getting to him on our first night in Zemio, somehow sleeping through the noisy rain that should have awakened him. He attributed this to doxycycline, which is not known to me as a hallucinogen as other antimalarials can be. I thought I would help by telling him a story about the OR in Banda. We had been operating at two tables. The nurse put her hand out to the Mayo stand next to the window to grab an instrument and picked up a green mamba instead! It had crawled though the louvers of the window and onto the sterile tray and its instruments. Sounds like an apocryphal story, right? Or an overdramatization of daily life in central Africa?

Ask Bruce. He was lagging behind us on the morning of that third day. We were already at the theater when he came rushing in with tachycardia and his hair standing on end. In his stroll over from the main house to the theater, he happened upon a snake in the middle of the path—and not just any snake, not just an innocent, I-am-trying-to-get-out-of-your-way garden snake. It was a cobra, and a spitting cobra at that. It reared up and assumed the striking pose, focused on Bruce. Spitting cobras aim for the eyes, since cobra venom can be absorbed through the conjunctiva. Bruce was already running backwards to get away, and paused only long enough to get a far-off telephoto shot of his assailant. Accosted by the flash, the snake slithered away into the grass. Ambroise said that Bruce should have screamed like a woman in distress and the men of the compound would have rushed over to kill it. This is a good explanation, I said, of why the people here go to such daily effort to machete off every bit of grass within ten meters of their houses or doors or windows or walls, scorch the earth in a protective moat around any settlement, and sweep fallen leaves from their dirt floors each morning.

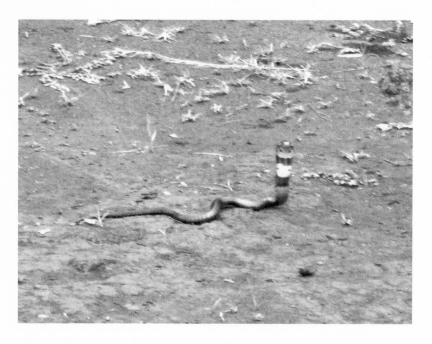

Bruce's spitting cobra, which gave him palpitations on his walk to the clinic.

But Bruce's encounter with spitting death couldn't dampen the other highlights of the morning. First, during our post-op rounds at six o'clock, we found big smiles and blessings upon us from all sides, even from those with recently closed wounds. Biggest of all came from the fellow with the massive hydrocele, who'd had his scrotum torn apart with just a bit of local anesthesia.

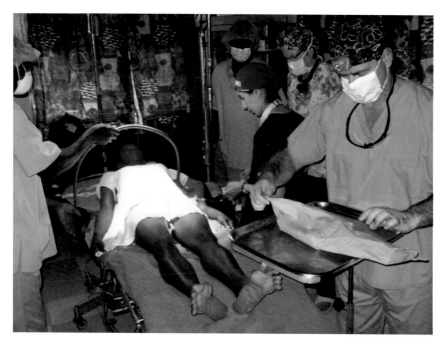

The team in Zemio preps one of our ovarian cyst patients. We see many female patients with long-untreated cysts and benign tumors of the uterus during these missions.

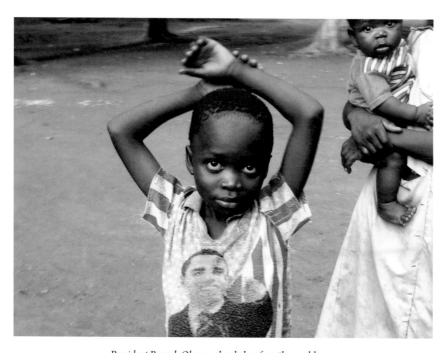

President Barack Obama clearly has fans the world over.

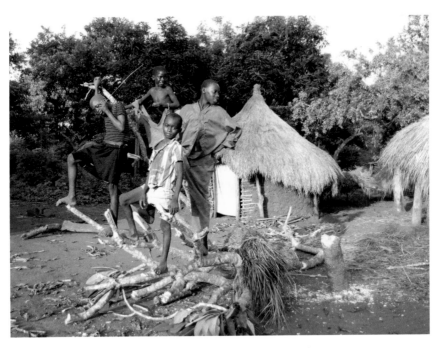

Young Zande boys in the settlement of the Assa refugees.

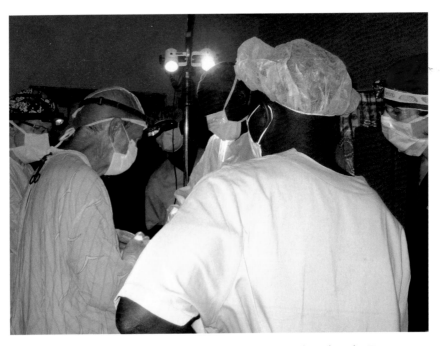

All hands were on deck to assist in the first-ever prostatectomy to be performed in Zemio.
It is likely that the only place where one could get a prostate operation
in the whole of CAR was in the tiny mission village of Zemio during our visit.

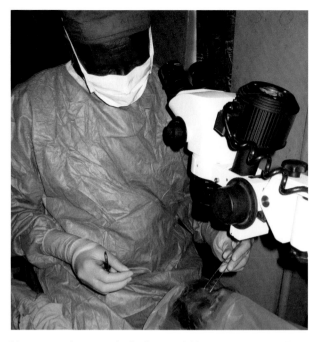

One of the very, very few pieces of technology available in Zemio is a surgical microscope used by Ambroise Soungouza for cataractectomies.

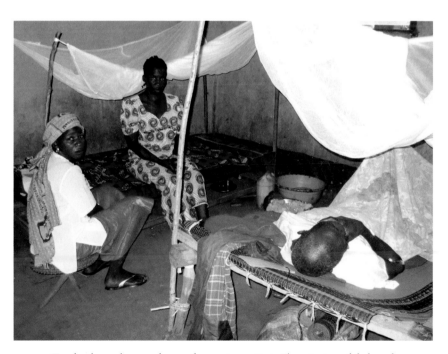

Two family members care for one of our post-op patients. The patients are fed, cleaned, and clothed by family members. There are no nurses or orderlies to offer such care.

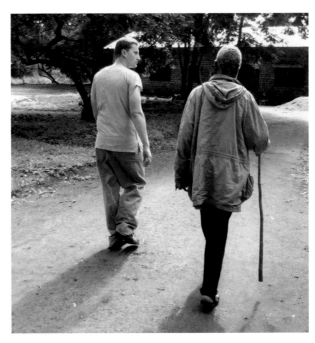

Josh walks a post-op patient, who is using a walking stick, to the clinic for a final checkup. Early ambulation is a fact of life here, and a key to our good outcomes.

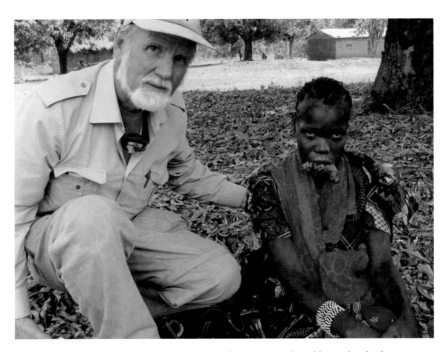

Our legendary patient, Flore. Her tumor was fast growing and would cause her death in a matter of weeks if we didn't take extreme action. Despite the challenges, we took Flore out with us to Kijabe, Kenya, where she could get the surgery and care she needed to survive.

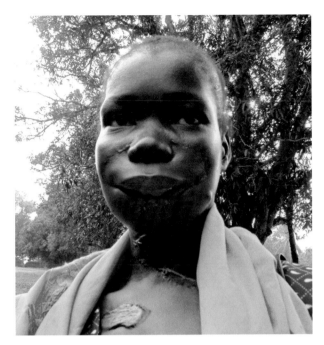

Flore post-op, with a functional result. Oral continence has been restored, so she can eat and prepare food. Though still shy, Flore is now caring full time for her five young children.

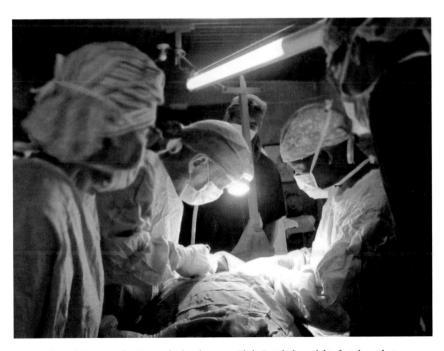

US Special Forces medics Dys and John observe as I help Isaiah through his first thyroidectomy.

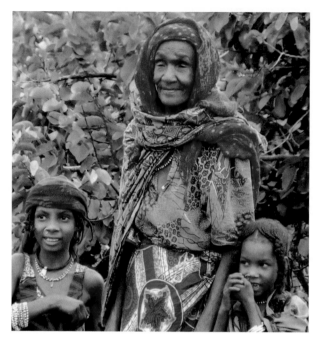

Mbororo woman with her children in Zemio, along the hajj route from west Africa.

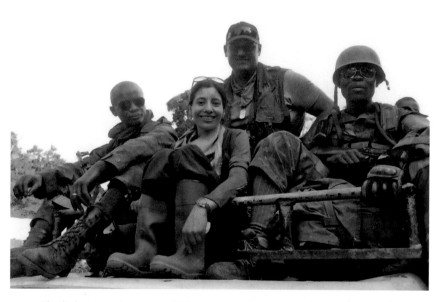

Claudia hanging out among our CAR army escorts during our rainforest road trip to Obo.

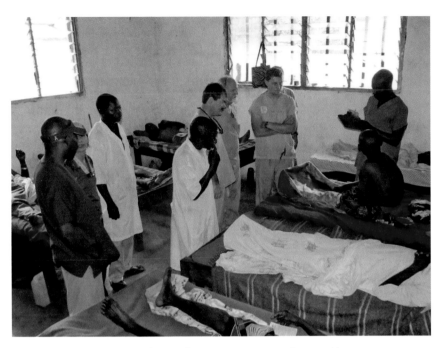

*Post-op rounds on our burgeoning inpatient population in Obo,
which set all records in the village's infirmary.*

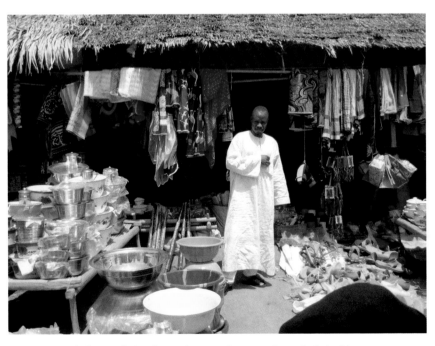

*With the arrival of Arabic-speaking, non-Bantu merchants, the look of the town
Mboki has changed. It now looks more like a village in the Sahel.*

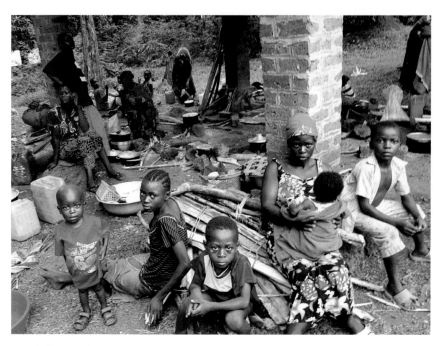

The "Diet Kitchen" in Obo. This is the caregivers' quarters, where food is prepared for inpatients.

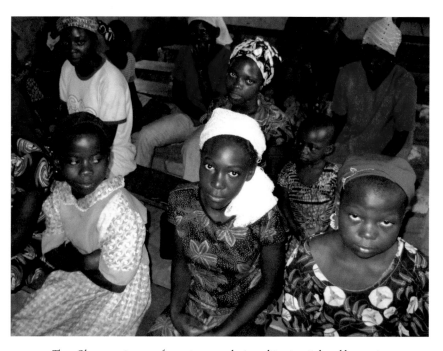

These Obo youngsters sang for my tape recorder in multipart, antiphonal harmonies.

And the woman who had had the hysterical reaction to ketamine on our first operating day? She was sitting very serenely in her bed, discussing things rationally with her family. She remembers none of her operation. No permanent harm was done.

We went back to the main house for breakfast, listening to children sing and pray at the beginning of their school day. I recognized one or two as the hymns that our young goiter patient had serenaded us with in Pazande. The songs of the Assa refugees are done in a call-and-response rhythm, with a foresinger leading off and the others following.

A few hundred meters from the Zemio station is another refugee settlement of Zande people, though these are not from Assa. This is the DRC mission station, and it is actually bigger than the Zemio station and also has its own Bible school. While the Zemio Bible school uses French and Sango (primarily for written materials) and Pazande (for most speaking), the DRC Bible school uses the Congolese language of Lingala, which was first reduced to writing, called Bangala, by the missionaries of the Summer Institute of Linguistics and Wycliffe Bible Translators. The DRC station also maintains its own time zone and is thus an hour later than all its surroundings. That's why you can hear the same song to start the day at each of the schools, sung in two languages, an hour apart—but from their perspectives, at the same time of day!

A special treat was being prepared for breakfast. Last night was the second night after a heavy rain, a typical time for the emergence of swarms of termites. The well-known termite holes around here are owned properties, and everyone knows who holds what rights to a given hole. No one can poach at the fleeting magic moment of emergence, which only lasts for about ten minutes. The locals can usually predict when that moment is coming. Last night at about ten o'clock was that moment. A number of kids spread throughout the community to stake out their holes, and there they waited for the phenomenon—a rather spectacular show. The hole in the ground becomes a buzz from which a winged horde flies up on its maiden and nuptial flight. The wings fall off like detachable gliders shortly after the flight begins; they're designed only for mass movement in the mating swarm, which will not happen again until the next big rain. The flying termites have to be captured quickly, but they take to the air by the hundreds of thousands from each hole, so they are easy to catch (yet many millions escape and keep the cycle alive). The little kids gathered them by hand and bucket. In very little time they had filled a five-gallon *bidon*, or old jerry can.

Thus was breakfast provided: We received a small bowl of roasted, high-protein wingless termites. Mary Anne Harris said, "I do not know anything that does not eat the termites—birds, big and small beasts, and all Africans, with the one possible exception being white people from America." Still the hordes get enough survivors through. We didn't want to be apart from the Africans in their feasting, so we each had a small sample of roasted termites for breakfast. They have a kind of scratchy, nutty taste.

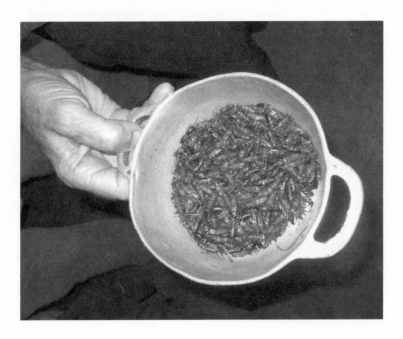

*A bowl of tasty roasted termites—a special treat after
the rains spurred a great termite mating flight.*

After the excitement of the morning, we headed into another full day in the OR, with a side goal of trying to cement our plans for getting to Obo— or not.

We had spent time over the last couple of days and in the mornings training the nursing staff in order to get them comfortable with the through-and-through irrigation to clear clots in the catheter and get good urinary outflow for the patient with the enlarged prostate, the man who had to undergo bladder puncture several times a day. This was the day for his prostatectomy.

The nursing team was eager to have a go, and so was Ambroise, who was hoping that I would show him how it is done. He had not done a prostatectomy—this was his *première fois*, his first time. Our own team had not seen such a procedure except at a rather respectful distance, and the indigenous group needed to learn it as well. And so we began. As incredible as it may seem, we were undertaking a prostatectomy, entering just above the pubis and through the bladder, without any of the "necessary" tools for cauterization or suction, without a three-way catheter, and without any of the urological instruments or sutures or lap sponges to hold urine and blood.

I took Josh VanderWall through his first spinal anesthetic. We injected the bupivacaine and the fellow was ready with a little ketamine anesthesia preceded by an atropine prep.

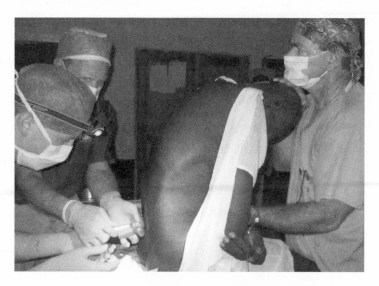

With Bruce and I assisting, Josh helps perform his first lumbar puncture, creating an effective block for our prostatectomy patient.

I guided Ambroise through his first Pfannenstiel incision, the type of incision usually used for a Cesarean section delivery, and then went through the fascia at the midline, splitting the muscles, entering into the blood vessel–filled space where the bladder lives. The thick detrusor muscle, a layer of the bladder wall, was incised between stay sutures, and then we entered the bladder. We had to use a laparotomy pad to absorb any urine in the bladder since no suction was available. So far so good.

I felt the bladder neck and the prostate. The patient had lateral lobes that were not greatly oversized; the obstructing part was the median lobe. That was a problem. Getting the median lobe out would be tricky and would probably require dismemberment of the bladder and urethra, with all the potential hazards of having to put in a critical life-saving device (a traction Foley catheter) that would require constant nursing care, or even cutting apart the muscles of the bladder neck (a Y-V plasty) to relieve obstruction from the hypertrophied detrusor muscle of the bladder wall. I began to wonder whether it would be a good idea to encourage the local team to attempt this kind of operation when the urgency that had brought us to do this operation was urinary retention, which might be solved by simpler means. Since he was puncturing, we could relieve that by a suprapubic cystostomy, which involves placing a catheter through the skin just above the pubic bone and into the bladder. Over time, scar tissue builds up around the catheter, creating a channel. Every so often, the catheter would have to be replaced, but it would allow him to urinate without the hazards of a big resection of the critical median lobe.

We moved forward with the plan to add to the Mayo stand two Foley catheters and a red Robinson catheter (made of rubber), hoping we might be able to introduce the Robinson catheter from inside the bladder neck, threading it out through the penis, or use some catheter-stiffening agent, like a Bakes dilator, as a probe to go from the outside in through the swollen prostate. However, we lacked equipment and could not get the flexible Foley catheter in the urethra—showing the high degree of obstruction—nor could we pass the Robinson catheter down through the bladder neck and out the urethra. If we could have, we might have tethered the Foley catheter to the Robinson catheter and pulled it back up inside. We tried each direction repeatedly and could not make it work, and we had no stylus that would allow us to make the turn through the prostate from either direction.

We had to stop the operation. In a moment, I had an idea and asked Josh to run back to the main house and get a coat hanger I had packed in my bag. He ran back with it as we waited. We bent it into a loop, creating a make-shift stylus. With no sterilizing solution except the Betadine, we dropped it into a bowl of iodine and after a minute of surface exposure threaded the Foley catheter over this coat-hanger stylus and then guided it through the prostate, through the perineum, and into the bladder. Now we had a large channel outlet from the bladder and could resect the median and lateral lobes of the obstructing prostate. We hyperinflated the Foley catheter balloon and used the inflated balloon to tamponade the bleeding surface of the bed of the resected prostate. With the Foley catheter pulled down for traction to achieve hemostasis and the lumen of the catheter as an outlet for urine and irrigation fluid, I placed a second Foley catheter through the abdominal wall and into the bladder to use as the irrigation inflow, the suprapubic cystostomy catheter.

We sewed the catheter in place and closed the bladder in three layers, as I was once accustomed to doing as a renal transplant surgeon. In a week or ten days, the local team might remove the urethral Foley catheter and still have the security of the cystostomy tube. If they clamp the tube and hydrate the fellow to see if he can urinate, and he does, they can keep the cystostomy tube clamped for another month and then simply remove it once he is peeing normally and the channel has healed. He should never have to puncture the bladder again.

At the end, I turned the case over to Leenta, who now had the thrill of suturing the skin closed—operating all alone, though she had only put in her first skin suture yesterday. And I am happy to report that the irrigation routine worked well with the nurses in the infirmary and that the fluid return was clear and without clots.

Première fois all around! But not, I might add, the first time I've used a coat hanger as a surgical tool. We did many more operations throughout the day—all important, but none quite so dramatic.

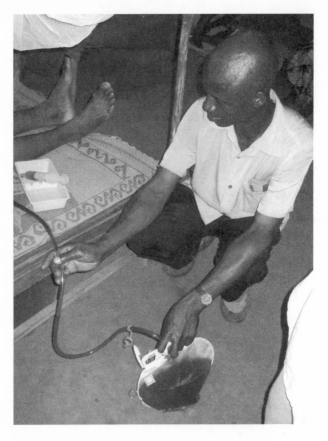

Bienvenue carefully watches the still-bloody catheter line from our prostatectomy patient.

In consultations, we saw a relatively young man—whom I will call Pascal—for a problem unusual for his age. He was well dressed, sporting a soccer club's T-shirt, and rumor had it that he drove here in a small vehicle—a rarity. We discovered that there were two reasons that Ambroise wished for us to see him: to potentially solve *his* problem, and to potentially solve *our* problem.

Pascal's problem was one of dysphagia (difficulty swallowing) and a series of fevers. When you see recurring fever here, malaria is the first thought, but he was on artemisin-based antimalarials. As we talked with him, we discovered that he was experiencing weakness and weight loss, but that could have been due to the difficulty swallowing and not a primary problem. A quick look at his throat revealed what appeared to be thrush, or candidiasis, a fungal infection. We had antifungals, so it was treatable, but as always, we had to ask the question: Why should a young and healthy-looking man have a disease that is usually an opportunistic invader of immunocompromised patients? He anticipated the question by pointing out that he had tested negative for HIV a week before. He was not taking either steroids or other antibiotics. We switched him to doxycycline and co-trimoxazole, both active against the malaria protozoan parasite, under the assumption that he might have one of the strains of artemisin-resistant malaria now being reported in the region. Then we had to wait and see.

Having attended to his problem, we got down to our business and asked not what we could do for Pascal but what he could do for us! We had been asking many sources if there might be a vehicle near Zemio suitable for transporting us to Obo and had learned that there were only two vehicles nearby, each of questionable roadworthiness, particularly during the rainy season. Pascal represented the owner of one of the vehicles. He was the driver of a small, ancient Toyota truck with welded steel racks on top of the cab and rails welded along the sides of the bed to accommodate a large load. Our chariot awaits?

We began negotiations, first for the cost of fuel and then for the length of the drive and the number of people to be carried and the payload. It looked like a grand adventure—overland to Obo! Right! We needed some further information, including what supplies were available here for us to carry or in Obo for us to use and the cost of an armed security escort. There were seven of us, and we would take four of the staff from the Zemio station—Ambroise, Isaiah, Sacco, and Celestine—leaving the others to cover the "call" here. That would be eleven, not counting the driver and the escort. I had hoped we could leave our personal gear in Zemio and divide drugs and surgical equipment among our packs. Perhaps half of what we had brought in would go with us and much of that would not return. But we would need several pieces of equipment that they did not have in Obo, where conditions are far more "rustic" than they are here. We would need the sterilizers, the generator, fuel, lights, instruments, and the "software" that goes with them—gowns, gloves, sutures, skin preps, etc. The load was growing.

We looked at Pascal's truck: It was a well-kept but ancient and often-transplanted machine. The tires were well worn and I could see no spare. When I looked more closely at the outer wall of the tires, I saw that two of them had holes or tears that had been sewn up. When I looked closer, I thought I recognized 2-0 Vicryl sutures in the tire casing!

I asked the driver how long it might take to get us the seventy miles (as the hornbill flies) from here to Obo. "It depends on the rains," he said. "It has taken three days." I did not believe that was the kind of adventure at the pole of inaccessibility that we had come for, particularly given the investment. We needed to make good use of every hour, so I was hoping to make it there in less than a day, even on the rainy-season road. But who could estimate how bad the roads might be?

And, of course, we have potential Lord's Resistance Army activity along that stretch of road. A convoy filled with innocents with cash and valuable surgical supplies would be ripe for the picking and would be short work for anyone interested in picking up a few hostages. We would need two soldiers of the Central African Republic army, a few of whom were stationed at a small base near the Zemio airfield. If we engaged them, it would be the biggest deal they would ever negotiate with the only solvent entity in the area. Like the soldiers in most of the countries in central Africa, they usually just forage in the countryside and "live off the land"—or the people who inhabit it.

The driver quoted me a price in Central African francs, at an exchange rate that was anyone's guess. Ambroise said he could make the currency exchange if we had greenbacks. It would be US $750. What I got through translation is that the driver's small truck might be adequate to hold the medical supplies, but would be inadequate to hold the twelve personnel and whatever personal supplies we would need until AIM AIR flew into Obo to pick us up five days later. Pascal said he would check to see if a Toyota Land Cruiser might be available; they often materialize when an American happens by. We would have to negotiate again for a second vehicle, and possibly even a third. As we added vehicles, we'd have to increase the number of armed escorts who rode along with us, making it even more likely that we would need the third truck, if only to help carry our security. Although no one yet knew anything about the availability, cost, and carrying capacity of multiple vehicles, they were eager to negotiate with US cash–carrying parties.

I said we would shoot for a Sunday trip with a decision on whether it was a go or a no-go by Saturday evening. We would wait to hear more, especially from Mark Pearson, who was trying to make contact with the Uganda People's Defence Force folk who are often flying overhead, burning fuel subsidized by the United States just to show the flag, and putting in air time for credit in future job applications. There is certainly no humanitarian service being provided by that group, as their ultimate refusal to transport us into Obo in 2011 revealed. That service, apparently, is my responsibility.

I keep being reminded that the kinds of illnesses and required drugs and excessive pill consumption of the average "metabolic syndrome" patient in the United States may be the coming plague in Africa. The kinds of illnesses they could not possibly afford before—obesity, hypertension, diabetes, and depression—are getting to be more common here. The GERD (gastroesophageal reflux disease) medication I had overstocked on my trip here a few months ago is now all used up. Throughout the day, a couple of medical problems were resolved with drugs that I was told the day before we did not have. In fact, they did not have them until we arrived and restocked them, although they still had some of the drugs and surgical supplies I had left in Entebbe in 2011 to be forwarded to them and some that I had stocked six months before.

The pressure to keep supplying medications and expertise and training doesn't let up. A Zemio pastor came in with a chronic problem, which he is managing for the time being but wants to be rid of: rectal prolapse. When he has a bowel movement, the mucosal part of the rectum falls down and comes through the anus. It might require a rectopexy, in which we would tack the colon inside to the pelvis sidewalls. Most surgeons in the developed world would treat this by simply doing a sigmoid colon resection. That, however, would require a bowel prep and a several-day hospitalization in which he would need to be monitored, and that is too high a risk in this environment, which is less than adequately sterile and where the patient care is rudimentary.

I told them that this pastor should follow conservative therapy, using sitz baths and deworming medication (as intestinal worms can be a cause of this problem). We will check back with him on a future mission. Ambroise then pointed out that the next mission should include surgical care visits to Mboki (which lies between Zemio and Obo) and to Jonglei Province in South Sudan, and do not forget Am Timan, Chad. Of course. He had just described a quarter million dollars in air transport and six to eight weeks for each successive mission at several thousand dollars a day. "You know that I'm not a UN agency, right?" I asked. He summarized the conversation by saying, essentially, next time, we will do the pastor, and that will be soon—the same statement I had heard repeated to other patients.

And yet sometimes, a solution is easily and affordably offered. A large woman came in for a classic "limp in, leap out." She was obviously in pain and had an awkward gait, using a walking stick as she leaned to one side. There was a problem with her hip, she said. Sure enough, a hollow space had developed on her thigh, which she said had been present for the past three months, although it had happened to her before. I guessed she had a congenital hip dislocation and was now in anterior dislocation. Ambroise determined that she should have analgesics, since we had nothing further to offer. In terms of total hip replacement, that was true. But an operation isn't the only option, and often not the best option.

I asked her if she could lie down on the floor. She spread out her cloth and lay down. I lay down next to her on my back and showed her what I was going to do to her: I rotated my flexed right hip internally and abducted it by pulling my right heel over my pelvis. Then I helped her do the same, moving her leg manually through the position. Just as Bruce and Joe walked in, they heard the "pop." The woman stood up with a normal pelvis, no longer tilted. She left her stick by the wall and walked out smiling.

A few times we get lucky. And that idea made me think of my mother, who suffered from a congenital hip dislocation. Bruce and Joe were speechless as they watched this woman who had staggered in on a crutch. As she walked triumphantly through the queue of waiting patients, I said to her retreating back, "This one's for you, Mom!" Bruce and Joe turned to me with questioning looks, but I did not elaborate.

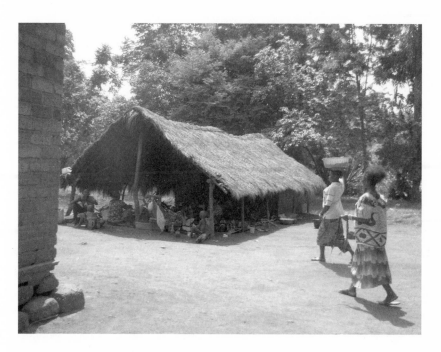

A thatched tent serves as the caregivers' quarters.

We actually came out before dark, in the late afternoon, and could do rounds to talk with the family members who were there as caregivers for the patients. That included the wife and brother and other family members of the prostate patient, all of whom were effusive in their thanks. All of the patients were doing well, though one hysterectomy patient had a fever. It was responsive to antimalarial medication, though, proving that here, malaria recrudescence is the most likely cause of post-op fever. There are four common causes of fever post-op in the developed world: wind (pneumonia), water (urinary tract infection from catheters), walk (deep vein thrombosis or vein inflammation from blood clots), and wound (an infection of the surgical wound). Walk is certainly a first-world problem, since many Western post-op patients are afraid to get up and move around. But here, patients are required to walk out of the OR unless they had a spinal anesthetic. Because we do so much operating under local anesthetic, we don't use catheters all that often. Early ambulation is the rule. As evidence, I pointed out to the team that there are no bedpans on this ward!

Here patients with post-op fever are first treated for malaria. With operation, injury, or childbirth, there is blood loss, and when the body experiences decreased blood volume, the spleen contracts in order to reinfuse reserved blood back into circulation (the spleen retains blood for just such a function). The spleen, as well as the liver and other splanchnic organs in which blood pools and circulates, also happens to be where the hypnozoites of Plasmodium falciparum (the parasite that causes malaria) doze. The use of these reservoirs injects these parasites into circulation, resulting in the classic shaking chill and fever of malaria recurrence.

We'd had an eventful day, but there was one more big accomplishment to attempt in the evening. When we arrived in Zemio we discovered that despite the new cell tower and the phone cards and services purchased in Entebbe, we had no connection to the outside world. Some locals occasionally had service, and it was a frequent topic of discussion—was the cell tower working and could you get a signal. It seemed that the cell tower ran on a generator, so would often be without power. Mary Anne had received one call on her phone but was convinced it was a gag, since the caller said "Joe's Pizza." Still, I was anxious to make a call. It was my grandson Matthew's eighth birthday.

Mary Anne Harris gave us the satellite phone for the mission station, to be used in emergencies, but it hadn't been used yet. We moved out from under the trees to a flat, clear space that had once been a tennis court (yes, a tennis court). We tried five times to get a satellite fix, but could get no reception. Well, we tried.

After putting away the satellite phone, we almost casually tried the cell phone one last time. On the first ring, it went through to Gainesville, Florida! It switched to voicemail and I left a fifty-two-second message, telling Matthew that this is Grandpa Glenn making a call from Zemio mission station, Central African Republic, to wish him a happy eighth birthday.

One more first for the day! It was something we contemplated as we walked out under the cloudless sky with golden weaver birds twittering in the palms and ficus around us and the long nasal-sounding honk of the hornbill. In the absolute and abrupt darkness of equatorial Africa, we spotted constellations in the multitude of stars, observed the cut edge of the Milky Way, and watched the passing Space Lab, a distinctive, oversized satellite moving in equatorial orbit. While space-age junk circulates above us, down here, near the pole of inaccessibility, we are reusing the castoffs from societies of redundancy for critical workarounds that have great consequence to human lives—and recycling an occasional coat hanger.

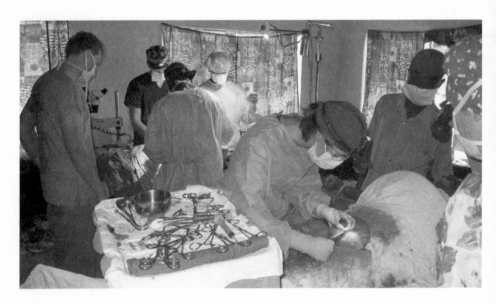

We kept two operating tables busy at all times. In the foreground, Leenta holds the torch while Claudia closes and Isaiah observes. On the second table, other team members are midoperation.

CHAPTER SIX

RESPONSIBILITY
AND RESOURCEFULNESS

June 8, 2012, Zemio mission station

I WAS UP EARLY AND MADE ROUNDS ALONE. AS I STROLLED OVER TO the infirmary, expecting an entourage behind me, I found that the team members had stopped for their ritual ceremonies around the totem coffee press that traveled with us. It gave me an opportunity to observe kingfishers calling for their mates in the canopy along the walk. At the clinic, I met up with Bienvenue, the nurse who had been caring for the prostate patient throughout the night. Bienvenue had been told of the gravity of the situation, the importance of maintaining the irrigation system and through-and-through flow of the catheters. He got the message. He had not slept, and he had carefully recorded the fluids in and out, which balanced perfectly and showed that we were not pumping in fluid that could have leaked into the retroperitoneal abdomen. The urine coming from the Foley catheter was a lemon yellow without a trace of blood, clots, or any other evidence of hemoglobin.

The staff had really taken to this higher level of responsibility and was proud of its critical work. When Bruce told Bienvenue that he should go home to sleep or at least take a nap while we were looking after the irrigation and catheter flow, Bienvenue refused, saying, "The patient and the family will know I have left, and I do not want them to think I abandoned them when you have told me how important this task is." Good for Bienvenue!

With such a good job done in the critical component of nursing care, which had previously limited the number of operations we could do on prostatic obstruction patients, we decided we could proceed with the next one. And the success of the cystostomy tube meant we weren't encouraging a heroic but foolhardy and dangerous resection that might turn bloody and result in a host of potential complications.

Jean Marco arrived that morning wearing a green-on-white floral-patterned shirt. I know that shirt well. It is Jean Marco's "come to meet Dr. Glenn shirt," his "Sunday go to meeting" shirt, which he wears because he knows he is going to have his picture taken with me. I pulled out a copy of *Out of Assa: Heart of the Congo* (Three Hawks Publishing, 2000) and flipped to a photo of Jean Marco and me at the airstrip at Assa. I am holding a spear, and he is standing next to me—wearing the green-on-white floral-patterned shirt. The photo was taken twenty-four years earlier, and he confirmed that the shirt is over thirty years old. I pointed out to the group that one of my friends had once bragged that he could wear the same size clothes he had worn in high school. "What do you mean?" I replied. "I still wear the same clothes I wore in high school!"

My discussion with Jean Marco resulted in a more realistic appraisal of the potential road trip to Obo. We had only made it there in the past via a thirty-minute, seventy-mile flight each way. And we were now in equatorial Africa in the rainy season. Under ideal circumstances, if we left very early, we might be to Mboki by noon and could conceivably arrive sometime after midnight in Obo. It is dangerous to drive at night in the rainforest given the potential for breakdowns and washouts, let alone LRA activity, which is why we had only gone by air in the past. We could lose several operating days just to be able to say we had also worked at Obo. We could not spend several days away from a critically valuable clinical schedule to stagger about on an uncontrolled trip. Further, we would have to dislocate all of our equipment, including generator and sterilizer, and only take a couple of people as our trainees, since we could not leave the Zemio station uncovered, especially in view of the hectic call schedule for emergencies and illnesses and post-op care. We would diminish the teaching role of the Zemio team in order to gain access to the patients awaiting services in Obo. Still, those patients were in need.

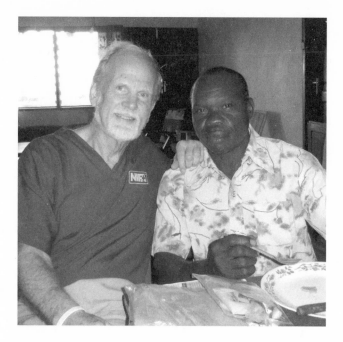

Jean Marco and me; he is my friend and guide from Assa, Democratic Republic of the Congo, who led the refugees into the bush and over the river into the Central African Republic.

So we awaited a response from Mark Pearson, who was investigating air transport. That option would render moot many of the objections to the hazardous, uncomfortable, uncertain, expensive, and potentially too time-consuming overland transit.

In the meantime, we had not run out of cases at the Zemio station, although many of our potential patients had been squeezed by the require-ment that they contribute a certain amount toward their care to cover the expenses of the infirmary and the clinical nursing staff. Potential patients who had been screened in consultation for elective operations but were unable to come up with the deposit for their care, as much as $20 for some, had returned to the refugee camps. Some patients with more urgent condi-tions were encouraged to come back to see what the doctor from America could do to pay for the operation. Of course, later I discovered that the costs I was expected to pay included everyone's. There might be a lesson for health-care reforms hidden somewhere in this discovery.

One of the important functions of the Mission to Heal trips is the performance of cataract operations. We had one scheduled for the fourth day, and for the first time in Zemio, we would use real cataract kits, which Ambroise had once seen used in Bangassou, a city of about twenty-five thousand people, 180 miles to the west. I refer to the style of operations we do as "cataractectomies under a tree." When Bruce asked me if we were going to do it with loupes, which are magnifying inserts in glasses for surgeons, I said, "How about this operating microscope?" We actually had a scope and a generator to power it. We had a large number of cataractectomy kits, but only twenty-five intraocular lenses. These were the first seen in this theater and would soon be transported to other areas served by the network of the indigenous church clinics.

We set up for the first cataract operations, which were very well done indeed. I observed while Ambroise was capably assisted by Emmanuel, who had been feeling like he was not being used at his full level of ability. As his reward for the good assistance, we made sure he did the next hernia repair.

The first cataractectomy was performed on a fully conscious man. The stay sutures to retract the eyelid were placed before the topical anesthetic—a bit of a stress test, more for the observers than the patient, it seemed. The lid retractor was inserted and the operating microscope was moved into position over the patient. It seemed almost pointless to have carefully donned scarce gowns and gloves when we were turning the unsterile, uncovered knobs of the microscope by hand. There were no foot pedals, as there are in Western operating rooms, so every adjustment to the microscope was a violation of sterile technique. As usual, though, necessity dictated.

The man's eye was held open and a bright light shone down upon it— about the only advantage of having a cataract is that without the cataract, the focused light is painful. Soon we were in the process of taking out the clouded lens. The conjunctiva, the outer covering of the eye, was peeled back on the upper edge of the iris. A small, handheld, battery-powered cautery tool, only big enough for these operations, was used to keep bleeding to a minimum, and a drop of topical anesthesia was dripped in while a syringe of lidocaine was injected into the retrobulbar space—the space behind the eyeball—to anesthetize all parts of the eye and to prevent the patient from moving the eye during the operation.

A small blade and small irrigating syringe were used to break any adhesions of the anterior lens surface to the interior surface of the cornea. As soon as this was done, the clouded lens could be slipped out, and almost immediately one of our rare and precious intraocular lenses was slipped into its place. We irrigated the area so the lens would remain seated while the microscope was used to make the ultrafine suturing possible. Only three stitches were needed to complete this simple and successful operation. A few drops of a topical antibiotic were placed in the eye and the stay sutures were unclamped. Then we placed a patch to keep his eye stationary and avoid the cornea getting scratched by any foreign material in the conjunctival sac, like blood, gauze, or sutures.

As Ambroise and Emmanuel were removing their very hot gowns, I guided the patient over to shake their hands; I didn't want him to identify me as the benefactor. Fortunately, the problem of patient confusion will be a nonissue when I am not here and these operations continue.

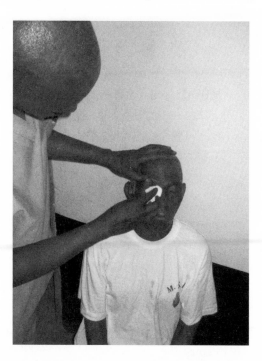

Ambroise removes the dressing from one of his cataractectomy patients.

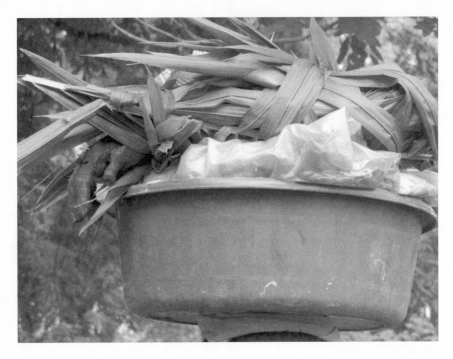

If you look closely at the left side of the container being carried by a woman from market, you will see a blackened hand protruding. In fact it is bush meat, or the hand of some primate, ready for the stew pot.

The consultations throughout the day were at least as interesting as the operations. Our first patient was the *chef du service*, or head, of the Médecins Sans Frontières (MSF)/Doctors Without Borders clinic in Zemio town, which began operating in the mid-1990s. They have permission from the capital to treat refugees in other parts of the country and use that as a blanket to also treat the Azande in Zemio. So we had the two medical chiefs of the area, Isaiah heading up Zemio mission station, and the Zemio MSF chef du service, both nurses who were in charge of their respective units. The man had acute right eye pain. Using fluorescein strip staining, we revealed a large corneal ulcer. I had told Josh many times that the only living tissue on the body that is visible externally is the cornea. All other surface cells are already dead or in the process of dying and being desquamated. The fluorescein stains dead cells, so it can be used in the cornea to identify damaged areas. The ulcer had the mapping of a viral infection, not the heaped-up edge of a bacterial infection. We treated him with a topical anesthetic and anti-viral and a topical antibacterial treatment, to be safe from superinfection of the ulcerated cornea. He said he was going to send us over a group of patients for tomorrow's operations. We would see if they arrived. I gave him my card and details to pass on to the MSF group, although I doubted that would make a difference.

When we had been in Zemio in January, we had met three MSF staff. They had sent a delegation to inquire about the rumor that someone was operating in Zemio. After introductions, one of our group suggested that he and an MSF staffer swap T-shirts, almost as a souvenir for each, and the response was a rather uncomfortable refusal: "Since this is our brand, we must all protect it." With some nervous clearing of throats, they said that they were here to assess health-care facilities and had heard that there were operations going on at the Zemio mission station. They followed this by saying, in a nondirect fashion, "We're the health-care providers here and we didn't authorize any such activities, so ..."

The unspoken censure hanging over the compound and our group brought silence with it. I did the talking for the team, describing the competencies and difficulties here. It was soon obvious that I was not a fly-by-night operator or a paramedic who had always wanted to cut someone open, that I had credentials longer than those of the whole MSF group in the CAR, and that my experience in the area had begun with this very group of people long before they were refugees. My talk was greeted with a lot of "Well, then." Given the tone of the initial meeting, I believed that they had come to say that they were the ones who should determine whether I should be operating, but we never got to that point. They realized how late it was and explained that MSF rules dictated that they return to the MSF base before dark. We had a patient who was ready to return to his family in one of the refugee camps, and I asked if they could carry him with them in their truck. No, they said, that isn't allowed. They said they would notify Brussels that they had met the operator and that he appeared to be a surgeon who intended to persist in his mission. They left, having been a bit short-circuited. And our post-op patient walked the few miles home.

I found a few minutes to type up some of the events of the day, a somewhat risky venture: If people see me sitting down with the laptop near the clinic, they assume that I'm bored and need something to do. Most nights I go to bed with a plan to write, but I struggle to keep my eyes open, even with the headlamp burning and the laptop propped up on my knees. So I needed to catch up and get the laptop charged by hanging around near the generator we use for the operating light. But in an almost Pavlovian response, a swarm of people usually came running, some from more than a kilometer away, when they heard the little motor coughing and clicking. This happened most of the time; people would be huddled up twenty-deep with their throwaway cell phones in hand, hoping to recharge them.

These charged cell phones might last a very long time, considering that nobody here buys a prepaid SIM card with more than fifteen minutes. Anything more than that takes a fair amount of wealth. Cell phones are cheap here, often free, but the prices of SIM cards are exorbitant. So cell phones here are still novelties, used to make the very occasional and very short call.

Joe also uses my laptop for downloading the video he has shot to achieve a kind of backup, which takes a toll on the battery. So I scramble at odd moments to record the memories and notes of this incredible experience, before one experience laps and overlaps with the next. But I had few moments before I needed to return to consultations.

On the morning of the fourth day, a mother brought in her three-year-old girl. The daughter had an interesting mark down the middle of her forehead and a lump on the back of her head. The mark was a sagittal hemangioma— a strawberry mark—extending right along the crest of her skull and over her head from occiput to forehead. I said to the team that she was lucky to have been born in such isolation. Had she been born in the West, doctors would have insisted that she get an operation done quickly, before the disease went away on its own, which hemangiomas often do. The birthmark was not causing her any problems and was gradually clotting off, scarring down, and remodeling, something kids do better than anyone else. "Neglecting" to treat it had been the best possible treatment. The only potential issue is that giant hemangiomas in the hands or extremities can be a sign of a disease that causes intravascular clotting. Blood clots form inside the blood vessels, consuming clotting factors the rest of the body may need, disrupting coagulation elsewhere, and causing abnormal bleeding throughout the body. This syndrome is called consumption coagulopathy type IIIa. When I asked to look at the girl's hands, which were clear, Ambroise actually knew what I was looking for. Zemio, apparently, isn't that isolated from the world.

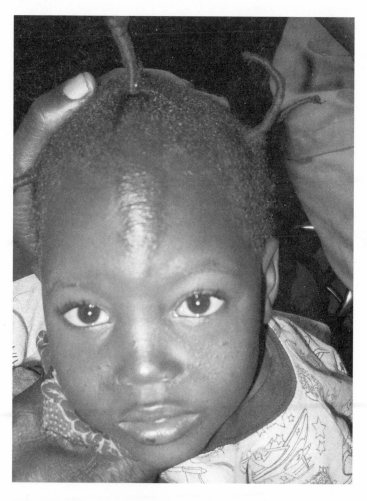

A young girl with a classic "strawberry mark" on her forehead. Here, there is nothing to be done. In the Western world, nothing should be done, yet it often is.

At some point in the morning, I was surprised to see the man with the varicocele, who had told us he had twenty-three children (a fact we found quite risible at the time). I had told him that he did not have the one indication I know of to remove it—infertility. But he was insistent and therefore came back to have it removed. Okay, fine, I said. It was a fairly simple operation. But what did our varicocele turn out to be? Not a varicocele at all, but a lipoma or fatty benign tumor—which makes the story of twenty-three children a bit more possible. And which goes to show that our diagnoses out in the jungle aren't always as accurate as they might be if we had more advanced diagnostic equipment. But of course, with more advanced equipment comes the expectation of more advanced procedures, procedures that are sometimes unnecessary, as the young girl with the hemangioma illustrated.

After we did a few consultations in the morning, the patient we had been waiting for walked into the theater. He had the classic appearance of a village elder, a serene dignity that implied he had weathered many problems and gotten through them all. His hypertrophic prostate was a real disability, and he needed a prostatectomy. We all hoped this would be a good teaching opportunity for the local team.

Dan inserted the spinal anesthetic, his first, with my help. This actually marked the very first case that was done entirely with the block of the spinal anesthetic—no local lidocaine injected in the skin and, best of all, no ketamine! With previous spinals, we had had to use one or the other in addition to the spinal, either because we needed to induce a more complete anesthesia or we needed a better local block. The patient was conscious and cooperative throughout the procedure, even when we were seeing if he could tolerate a self-retaining retractor and the stretching muscles to reach his bladder. It went well.

With this patient, the Foley catheter insertion was successful, after the balloon on the end had been tested by Claudia. Upon entering the bladder, I inserted a finger along the lateral lobes and could feel them swelling up on either side of the bladder outlet. This was the one to resect! The complex median lobe was not a major problem and the large lateral lobes could be removed by inserting a finger into a small incision and scooping them out with the curled finger. This was a perfect scenario for Ambroise to actually perform a prostatectomy. So, off to the races we went, and history may record June 8, 2012, as the opening day of prostate resection by the indigenous staff in the Zemio mission station.

I made a fingernail-sized slice in the bladder mucosa (allowing access to the layer around the prostate capsule) and had to restrain myself from simply scooping and shelling out the big lateral lobes of the prostate, which is somewhat easy after that initial dissection is started. *This is Ambroise's operation,* I thought, *and he should do it.* And so he did! We then began to blow up the balloon of the catheter—an important step since it is the downward pressure of the hyperinflated balloon on the torn bladder mucosa and the detrusor muscle of the bladder neck that controls the bleeding.

But the Foley catheter balloon would not inflate. It had been tested by Claudia, yet the catheter failed in its role at the moment it was needed. Blood was welling up in the bladder. Now what? Ambroise was going to pull the catheter out, but we would not be able to replace it by passing through the already torn muscles of the bladder neck. I took a large Vicryl suture and sutured the end of a new catheter (after its bag had been test-inflated) to the outlet of the failed one. Ambroise immediately recognized what was to be done and pulled the new catheter into the bladder, snipped the stitch, and disposed of the old, useless one. We inflated the balloon and pulled it down into the bladder neck, immediately slowing the bleeding in one of the inner layers of the bladder wall, the submucosa. Then we began the three-layer closure of the bladder and inserted the suprapubic cystostomy catheter as we closed the final layers. We hooked up the irrigation set and tried to irrigate from the cystostomy tube to get it to flow through the Foley catheter. It would run neither in nor out! I tried to clear the suprapubic cystostomy tube and it still did not work. Bruce got a Toomey syringe and saline and flushed the lower Foley catheter. A large clot was passed, and the fluid began flowing through. The irrigation was this patient's lifeline.

The deep chocolate brown of the bloody fluid through the catheter resolved after a bit of traction was pulled down on the Foley balloon, transforming it from pink to clear yellow. And no clots formed to block the flow. Score one highly successful inaugural prostatectomy at Zemio station!

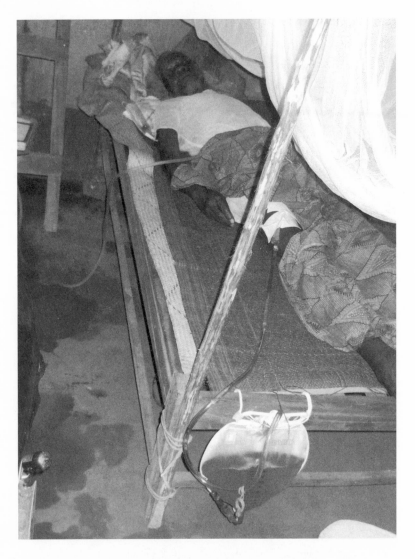

Our final prostatectomy patient, who walked over seventy-five miles to see us. Post-op, his urine cleared quickly to a cranberry color, without clots, thanks to a flow-through irrigation system managed by the nursing staff.

This was to be the last big case of our operating days in Zemio. I told the team we should not attempt another big case the next day, the day before we leave—*if* we leave. It isn't wise to attempt a complex case and then leave only inexperienced staff to manage the complications that inevitably result from "one-off" operations.

We went to do the next consultation in the OR antechamber. And what does the next patient have as he staggers in through the door? You guessed it! This elderly man had walked over seventy-five miles to get to us, dribbling about fifteen milliliters of urine every hour from overflow incontinence. He had urinary retention but no one to relieve him of it. The distended bladder could not contract against the obdurate obstruction and was simply dribbling urine out of the constricted pathway. He had come a long way as fast as he could manage with a considerable disability. Could we explain to him that because of a professional reluctance to leave any potential complications to a team that was by now rather well versed in how to manage the drainage system (and was in fact probably now at the peak of its expertise, having been freshly trained), he should just sit and suffer until a potential return visit—which was as yet unplanned? No, we couldn't.

Our bigger operations were taking consecutively less time, and we were getting more cases done in a shorter period. We hoped to get through the list of operations before our reserve of sterile supplies and disposable equipment—like gauze, gloves, and sutures—ran low. But on this day, we completed our list of patients by midafternoon, while the sun was still out—amazing! On our post-op rounds, we usually staggered around in the dark recesses of the infirmary to examine incisions under headlamps, but not on this day.

The family members of the prostatectomy and cataract patients were overwhelmed with gratitude. I suggested that the glory be directed to God, since we are just ancillary to a healing process we do not direct. Mary Anne Harris had come to visit the infirmary. She explained that she was not part of the operations since she was more oriented to the care of souls. I pointed to the bottom of the feet of a fellow whose hernia we had repaired earlier, noting the elephantiasis of one of them. It was clad in a size-sixteen sandal with a string that would allow it to adjust as the foot grew larger. I said that I shared Mary Anne's concerns but that one of my principal fields was the "care of soles."

With our patients well cared for by the nursing staff, we headed out to enjoy a brief exploration of the Zemio mission station and, excitingly, a visit to the Assa refugee settlement, a fifteen-minute motorbike ride away, not far from the Zemio airstrip.

I had learned that the LRA had come in three waves over Assa. The first two times, everyone fled, and this opened the village to the rebels, who took what they could carry. The third time, though, a group stayed behind to protect the village's residual belongings. This time the rebels captured those people and killed four. The rest were carried away as porters into the bush to experience who knew what horrors. Some of those who had been abducted by the LRA and escaped reported being forced to do everything from performing menial chores to beating other abductees to death to becoming sex slaves. Yet of all those who had been abducted, all but four returned. They are presumed dead.

Of course, the Assa refugees had lived through constant upheaval for years before being run out of their homes by the LRA: Hutus had fled into their region after orchestrating a Tutsi genocide in Rwanda and then losing control in the civil war. The northeastern Democratic Republic of the Congo is now the central location of the Hutu-Tutsi conflict. The DRC was plunged into civil war in the mid-to-late 1990s, and Laurent-Désiré Kabila overthrew the thirty-year despotic rule of Mobutu Sese Seko (whom we had seen immortalized in a memorial stone in Arua, Uganda). And then, just four years later, Kabila was assassinated by one of his bodyguards. This unstable "democracy" (called by some a "prefailed state," like the new South Sudan) does not control all of its sovereign territory.

In November 2011, there was an election in faraway Kinshasa, but the opposition leader (as well as many in the international community, including Secretary of State Hillary Clinton) called the results into question. Some of the Assa refugees had already returned, but it was feared that they would be disrupted again by civil war. My friends here in Zemio had intended to go back to the DRC soon, but rebel groups in the eastern DRC, still disputing the elections, had made travel unsafe. Of course, while the DRC has posted military units to protect villages in the eastern provinces from rebels, local peoples often feel that the country's own national army poses a greater threat to them than to outside invaders. The army has no infrastructure or supply lines, so troops forage off the populace as they move. (As of this writing, the United Nations has sent in troops to help end the conflict, but the rebel group M23, purportedly backed by Rwanda and Uganda, has stated that the UN has chosen to wage war on people who demand good governance.)

Still, the DRC refugees have their own Bible camp and are keeping their Pazande language and their time zone, assuming they will be allowed to go home when the office of the United Nations High Commissioner for Refugees (UNHCR) lets them return to the "pacified" areas—pacification largely resulting from the LRA's own mysterious planning, not from expulsion by an armed force of the sovereign state. Already, some from the Assa community had returned home or were going on scouting trips to see if it was safe. They had missed the planting season before the rains came, though, so they would have little to return to in terms of food, and if they returned, the UNHCR would stop offering support, as they would no longer be refugees.

In the Assa refugee village, gardens have been planted with cassava, squash, yams, and peanuts in an area previously considered too rocky to cultivate. The industrious Zande refugees carted in whatever soils they could find and started to plant and cultivate around the rocky outcrops before beginning the classic slash-and-burn ("swidden") technique. This is clearly not sustainable over the long term, but they were refugees hoping to return to the Congo, where their cultivated gardens are enriched with bat guano and other soils.

The UNHCR was needed for little here other than providing the peanut plantings and some food, though the agency is used to desperate, leader-less refugee peoples who cannot feed or house themselves. None of that was the case with the resourceful people of Assa. They have an almost perfect clone of an Assa village set among peanut patches and a variety of fruit-bearing trees.

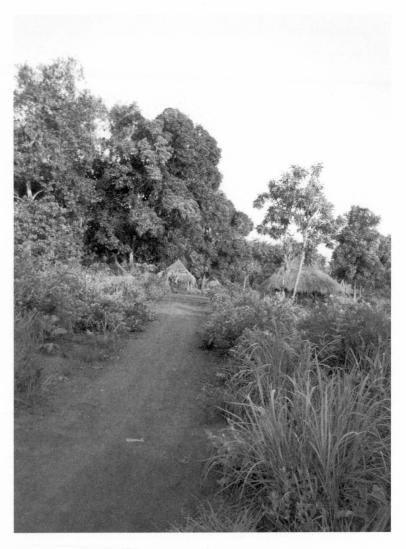

The road to the Assa refugee settlement.

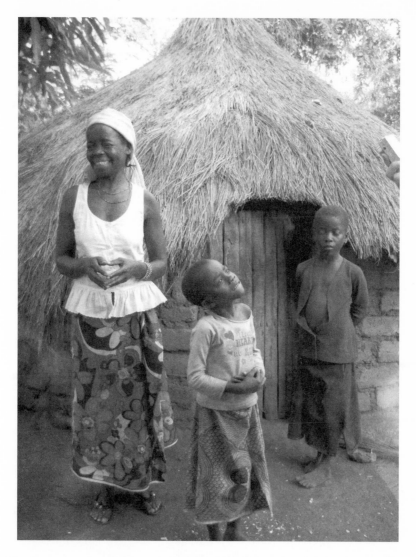

A Zande woman and two children in front of their thatched-roof home in the camp of Assa refugees.

Mary Anne had come with us to the settlement as our translator; she spoke both French and Pazande. I remembered all the Lingala greetings and could go along saying "*Bote mengi.*" While the people of Assa speak primarily Pazande, the market language of the DRC is Lingala, so they speak both. A couple of the older people knew me, and some of the younger ones had heard about me from the visit six months ago, if not from prior visits to Assa decades before. People were sitting outside to take advantage of the daylight to do their chores, such as mending nets for fishing for catfish and shucking palm nuts that they would press for oil, which they use for cooking. You can also make soap from these palm nuts, called "olives," hence the name Palmolive!

The scene seemed almost as peaceful as the ones I had seen in their home village in Assa. Their simple tools, the storage for their precious food stocks, their chickens, and a couple of goats are all here. It was a refreshing chance to stroll through *le vrai Afrique*—to see how the Azande sustain themselves despite all of the external turmoil that has befallen them.

We returned to the main house to have dinner and a good tutorial. We could overdose on pineapples and mangoes for dessert every day but we also had a special confection that looked like a double-ended bean. I held it to my upper lip like a Salvador Dali handlebar moustache while I explained that it is called *kouroukou* and is made of the mash left after the Azande extract the oil from peanuts.

I talked to Joe about his filming around the village during some of our operating time and asked him what he was planning with respect to a final product. He talked about a full documentary, and was hoping for a chance to go around with Les Harris to do interviews with several of the staff. He of course would need deep backgrounding before he could assemble B-roll and voiceovers, since he would need to capture the culture of these people as well as the distinctive culture of the missionaries and those like us who come to help in various ways. He had never heard of these people or this place, so he was innocent of what kinds of questions to ask or any context of anthropology or history in which to frame the interviews. He still had not discussed a time to interview me, which I thought curious.

During dinner, the cook hired by Zapai to take care of us during our stay placed a large plastic bottle of filtered water on the table in front of me and

Dan Vryhof, who incidentally had been manning the cook stove he had bought in Entebbe to sterilize the instruments. Dan filled both our water glasses and then took two sips, each time remarking how strong the kerosene smell was, looking around to see if it came from a kerosene lantern or the cook stove. Then he recognized the recycled water bottle—it had previously stored the kerosene he had been using to refuel the stove. Dan had a few good sips of kerosene-flavored water. I said that I hoped Josh, his roommate, was a nonsmoker!

Zapai, the local chief of the mission station, paid us a visit. He keeps everything running well and is the one who clears the airstrip and the roads and sees to all the housekeeping details like collecting payment for our room and board. He had come for an evaluation of his vision. He had impaired vision in his left eye because he was developing a cataract. He had good vision in his right eye but had the peripheral radial streaking of a cataract developing there, too, sort of like I do. He wanted advice and I told him that he should wait to see what happened with his right eye. If and when it becomes occluded, he should have them both done. Zapai was disappointed with that advice, but it was exactly what Ambroise had said to him earlier. He was eager to get them both done and move on. Nevertheless, I had Zapai stay on a bit. I still needed to work out a few things with him, including several of the housekeeping expenses of our stay as well as the AIM AIR bills.

Then—good news! Isaiah and Ambroise informed us that the road to Obo was in better shape than before because it had been graded, or leveled. That meant that the trip would not likely be more than a day. If we drove over to Obo on Sunday, we could operate in Zemio for a full day on Saturday, even adding that big case I had said I did not want to add. We would need Gilbert, another patient we saw and treated who is also the subprefecture commissioner, to rent us a Toyota Land Cruiser for the passengers. (Zemio is a subprefecture in the Haut-Mbomou prefecture of the CAR.) Les and Mary Anne had bought the used Land Cruiser in 1984, and it had been passed through several owners until it came to rest in the hands of the subprefecture commissioner. Along with the US $750 for Pascal's pickup, I had to somehow pay over a thousand dollars for the Land Cruiser in US currency that

Ambroise could convert to Central African francs. Or I could see if I could get AIM to cover the cost and debit it from my AIM account—which had a large number of charges floating on it already.

So we would let Gilbert know that the trip was a go. The two vehicles would be retained with a prepayment, and we could then load them with fuel. Ready? Now, stand in the bed of a truck with both hands hanging on to a steel bar and cover your eyes and head, since you will be swatted frequently with thick overhanging branches that threaten to wipe you off the truck altogether. Bend your knees to absorb heavy jolts and be prepared for a roller coaster ride as the vehicle slides through mud and dodges obstacles and washouts. This will be the ride to Obo, for seventy miles. Along with a host of unknown hazards, we will have to push the vehicles onto two ferries, hoping they do not slip from the muddy banks and into the river. We would have to have enough electricity in the camera batteries and the laptop to keep up to date on the photojournalism, but the bouncing around would prohibit any such work being done en route. After we arrive, if we are so lucky, we will have to be ready to go to work immediately, since we have little time in Obo to do what we had already been doing in Zemio.

We would pack up all our bags and stash them at the Zemio mission station hangar to be picked up when Jon Hildebrandt or another AIM AIR pilot stops in to get a couple barrels of fuel. We would have to let him know by cell phone that we would be in Obo for pickup and that since we have to go out from Zemio town for emigration, we would need to have him come to the Zemio mission station first to pick up our bags and fuel; the airstrip at Obo cannot accommodate us and our bags and an extra fuel load as well.

Amid all of this, the local team developed a new travel plan. Ambroise, Isaiah, Sacco, and Celestine would be going along, but they would not be returning with us. We would operate on as many patients as we could, but there would be more patients than we would have time for, and we hoped to save enough drugs and supplies to have the local team carry on for several days at Obo after Jon picked us up. Then the four of them would get the vehicles (with fuel supplied, of course, by their sponsor, *moi*) and come back slowly by road, stopping at many villages along the way to dispense care and even operate in Mboki (one of the sites proposed for the next trip of Mission to Heal). The big event of our trip will be our pass through Mboosa, the village where Ambroise was born—and where he would be returning as doctor and surgeon to the community.

I hoped that all of the contingencies would work out, because this is what we are doing here in the first place—indigenizing skills and working our way out of a job!

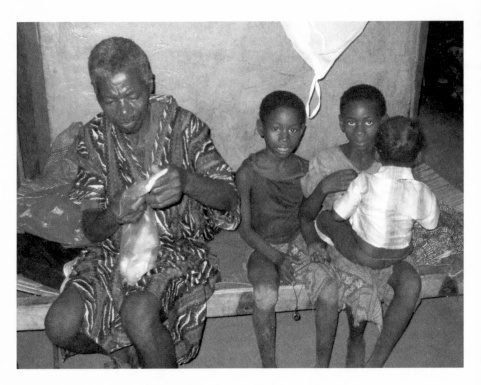

Family visiting hours for one of our recovering patients.

CHAPTER SEVEN

GIFTS FROM THE POOR

June 9, 2012, Zemio mission station

THROUGHOUT THE NIGHT, THE BIRDS WERE LOUDER THAN THE bats in their heavenly belfry for once. All night long the bats were hanging upside down on ripe mangoes, sampling each and trying to get away with a few. But over their chirping we could hear a few owls trying to sort out their marital status.

A little bleary-eyed after the long week, I walked over to the infirmary with the team the next morning to check on the patients. We looked on in amazement: All the patients were sitting up and raising both hands overhead in a salute and grateful greeting. Not one of the patients we'd operated on in our very busy week had any problems, and even those we treated late the day before were ready for discharge. They posed for portraits taken by Joe, usually with their hands raised heavenward.

The celebration stopped when I came around the corner into a separate room somewhat grandiosely labeled "Pediatrics." Lying on a wicker bed was a soundly sleeping baby of about ten months. He had been gurgling and cooing with a contented happiness when we saw him yesterday, and now he was sleeping soundly with milk on his lips. Next to him was his brother, about three, looking just this side of death. His mother stood in the corner against the wall with her hands covering her face—a mother usually knows when something big and bad is approaching her child.

The boy had severe pneumonia. His belly was protruding, and he was using every accessory muscle of respiration. I could see his intercostal spaces—the spaces between ribs—retracting. With every one of his very rapid breaths, he grunted, his nostrils flared, and his eyebrows arched up. He felt very hot to the touch.

I had seen him for the first time the day before. When he first came into the clinic, it was thought that he had malaria, so he was treated with Coartem. But he got worse. So we started him on amoxicillin by mouth. When I examined him, he had decreased breath sounds on the right side at the base of the lung and he was grunting and splinting—he would stop short in breathing in with each inspiration because of the pain. Yet he still put out his hand to shake mine with a frightened but subdued look on his face. When we had left the night before and made sure he was getting his amoxicillin, he was still splinting.

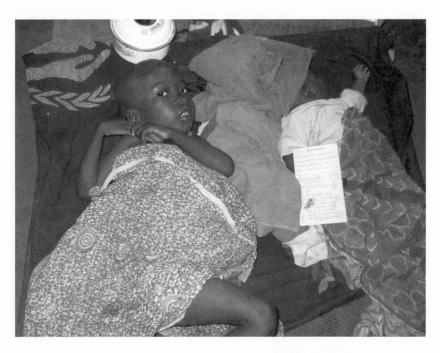

Our young pneumonia patient lying next to his baby brother,
who sleeps blissfully while his older sibling struggles to get enough air.

As we were going to the theater, I told our budding pediatrician, Josh, about the stages of progression in pneumonia. The first stage of consolidation brings on a "crisis" in which the patient either beats the disease or the "organizing" of the pneumonia occurs and the patient takes a turn for the worse. Our patient had turned in the wrong direction. He was wearing out from the work of breathing and his little heart was pounding so hard it could be seen banging against his anterior chest. His fever was higher than yesterday, and I could hear no breath sounds in the base on the right side. I gave him a couple of sharp slaps to see if we could clear this part of his lung, and we got a subteam to come back in and start him on an IV with a good dose of our second-generation antibiotic, cephalosporin. This kid needed help, and we were giving him everything we had.

We would have to wait and see. There was that uncertainty again.

I did more consults throughout the day, including the wife of Emmanuel and the wife of Isaiah, as well as one of Isaiah's five children, all of whom had the same problem—a resistant fungal infection of the scalp that had not responded to the antifungals the clinic had on hand. By happenstance, this was the first trip on which I had brought ketoconazole powder. The wives and all five kids got a head dousing of white powder as a way of controlling their tinea capitis. It made it easy to spot Isaiah's children when they were outside of the Bible school doing their military-like drills on the flat space that had once been the grass tennis court. They would line up, come to attention, and salute. A couple of them were even holding sticks, as if they were in the color guard or were carrying rifles. I think the goal was to encourage solidarity, if not paramilitary training, and to discourage them from becoming victims.

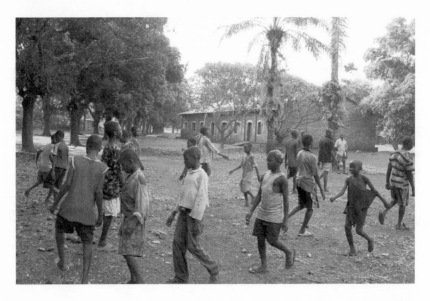

The boys from the Bible school march in the yard for their exercise. They look like cadets drilling as they march in a circle. I recognized one of my patients by the white antifungal powder on his scalp.

Two fellows came to see me, one with a large book. On opening it, I could see the compulsively drawn outlines of each tooth, the dental pulp, and its innervation. One of the men had made an atlas of the adult mouth in several color schemes and had a centerfold with a foldout of all the teeth, each of them numbered in their sequence. He wrote down his name and address and asked me for dental instruments, of which we had none, although we have had some on past trips. I promised I would see what could be requested and would show his pictures around.

The major—and only—operating case of our final day in Zemio deserved its special billing. After we saw several other patients, including a few more PID patients and a man with urethral stricture, I went into the theater to see our elder patient. He had worn his tattered but very warm "winter coat"—which doubled as a sleeping bag—on his long, slow, and painful road trip to the mission station. He still wore it as he walked into the theater. I couldn't help but consider the trip to Obo I had been negotiating. It was about the same distance, but in a vehicle, with guards, and with supplies—and yet still was being billed as uncomfortable.

I set up the spinal trays and lumbar puncture with Bruce, who would do his third spinal anesthetic of this trip, and of his life. This would be the second case in which we needed no local anesthetic or ketamine.

After the anesthetic was complete, I announced to the team that I would be out in the consult room and that Ambroise could call me when he wished to have me join. I wanted everyone to know that this was Ambroise's operation; he had mastered the Pfannenstiel incision and the preperitoneal approach to the bladder, which would be useful for other operations, such as bladder stones. This was the third time Ambroise had approached the bladder this week. In fact, we were doing sophisticated urologic operations, and considering that there are very few doctors in this country and almost no specialists, they likely aren't even being performed in Bangui, the capital. Miraculously, to be treated for lower urinary tract obstruction as a senior male in this nation, one would have to make his way to the remote mission station of Zemio!

As I waited in the next room, Ambroise opened the bladder and checked inside. Then he called me.

Something was different about this one. The patient had no really big lateral prostate lobes, but a very hard posterior mass, which seemed to be an obstructing median lobe tumor—and it was firm enough to be a cancer. We were not—and could not be—operating for cancer but to relieve urinary obstruction, which still required us to remove much of the mass. So we proceeded. It wasn't easy, but we got the majority of the median lobe grasped with the forceps and mobilized it up toward the bladder.

Ambroise was alarmed when he found that he had perforated the bladder, but it was a mucosal tear, which is part of the operation. We had to use that plane to get into the resection. When we had removed enough of the mass to unobstruct him, I had to decide whether to be content with that or to try to get the rest of it out. I figured as long as we had come this far, we might as well complete the resection, and we were able to remove almost all of the mass.

Bruce connected the inflow and drainage of the irrigation system, which he'd just taken from the catheter of our second prostate patient, who was doing well and no longer needed it, and we started the irrigation. Leenta was prepared to close the fascia and Dan to close the skin—but not until we investigated a mass in the patient's left groin. We opened it at the inguinal ligament and discovered that it was a hydrocele of the spermatic cord. Along the cord we saw several similar hydroceles and we excised them as well. Now the team could close.

I went over to see the successful post-op irrigation team in action after the patient was moved and discovered that the other patients, who had relatives all around, were adopting the third prostate patient. They were calling wives and brothers to bring fluid for him to drink, so he was surrounded by an entourage of helpers, including the basket-weaving brother of one of our other patients.

Transactions in Africa are rarely simple. Finalizing the convoy of vehicles and guards to get us to Obo required a series of complex negotiations and financial transactions with contracts and receipts in two languages. It took half the day, amid consults and our operation, and likely would have taken much longer if Les Harris hadn't been there to serve as scribe and translator. The cost had risen to $1,300 for the Toyota Land Cruiser. I had hoped to charge some of the costs to the account I use to cover the AIM AIR charges, an account that was already in the red. Gilbert, the Zemio commissioner, could accept an AIM credit, but Pascal needed cash. Oddly, unlike in Entebbe, Uganda, the people here aren't fussy about having the most recent printings or bills without the corners turned down. I quickly counted through my currency and found that I had $800 left. So I made a check out to AIM for Gilbert for the balance owed to him, Les wrote me a receipt, and Ambroise carried the check to Gilbert.

We urgently needed US currency to cover the fuel that must be purchased here and now for the several-week round trip. The distance is relatively short, but the vehicles aren't fuel efficient and the fuel is diesel. It costs $4 per liter, or $16 per gallon—four times what I would pay at home. The extended round trip would include Ambroise, Isaiah, and two other clinic workers, Sacco and Celestine. In Obo, they would handle simpler cases after we spent our time doing the more difficult ones and teaching them along the way. From there, the medical group would do consultations and operations at each stop on the return trip. The meds and surgical supplies we left for them would be well used along the road, and at each stop the status of these local Zande health-care practitioners would be heightened. When Ambroise returned to the village where he was born, he would do so proudly.

There were three "insurances" for the convoy of the two vehicles. First, one other fellow was traveling with us. Who was he? He "came with the vehicle." He was the onboard insurance policy, the traveling mechanic, the rental agency's agent, the overseer Gilbert sent along to see that the vehicles are tended to and used as indicated. He also "slept with the car"; in other words, he was the car alarm. His cell phone startled me when it rang; the ring tone was of a squalling baby.

The second insurance was my prepayment in cash and my access to the AIM account, along with my purchase of a burlap bag full of supplies and spare parts: extra oil, fuel, grease, and a "portable garage" that included tire patches like the ones already so liberally applied to the elderly tires of each vehicle.

The third insurance was the two CAR regular army guards in full battle dress (including uniforms, helmets, and AK-47s with multiple clips). For an additional $20 each per day, they would be riding on top of the ironwork over the truck cab, like those stagecoach guards you see in old Westerns. As I saw it, the principal use for their helmets was to protect their heads from the branch bashing they'd get as we drove through the rainforest; though, of course, they would still run the risk of being wiped off the top of the truck. I was fairly sure that the $40 per day would still have to be paid for all the days we kept the two guards out of the Zemio garrison, despite the fact that we would be dropping them at the Obo garrison for a week or so before they returned with the Zemio team on their weeks-long return circuit. Luckily, I could pay them out of my AIM account.

The CAR guard escort was necessary because LRA activity had sprung up along the road in recent months. During the week, there had been a killing by the LRA about sixty miles east of Obo. The LRA needs to carry out some random terrorist activity to show it is not intimidated by the concerted efforts of three groups on the prowl for them in the eastern CAR—the CAR army; the

Uganda People's Defence Force, sent by the African Union (composed of all African countries except Morocco); and AFRICOM forces, who were there to "reinforce intel and logistics" in what is diplomatically required to be an all-African action in the CAR. The AFRICOM website describes its mission as deterring and defeating transnational threats, preventing future conflicts, supporting humanitarian and disaster relief, and protecting US security interests. When we got to Obo, I would need to convince the battalion there to play that third role. I had my ways.

So to get this traveling road show underway, I parted with *all* of my US currency, without a source for getting more; checks, credit cards, wire transfers, and smartphones are nonstarters in this part of the world. The result was inevitable: Right after I surrendered the last of my money, I had other large bills to pay. Often a local would come to me demanding that I pay out twice as much as I had given him the day before, saying, "Well, you had it yesterday, so you certainly must have it today." In their eyes, all white men have a capacity to spontaneously generate great hordes of wealth, which seem to be rejuvenated each evening while they sleep. It almost makes sense if you consider the comparison between what they see me dispensing and what they have to dispense. But I could dispel that myth, and it was almost a relief to have parted with my last dollar, since all requests for more would get the same answer. And yet, some of the requests were for legitimate bills owed, such as the fee for our week of room and board, which I owed to Zapai. I owed $15 per day per person, and I believed I would owe a similar amount for our time in Obo. It would just have to await the arrival of the AIM AIR pilot, who could dispense cash that would be debited to my AIM account. My balance due would be sent to AIM's US headquarters, in Peachtree City, Georgia, and I would have to cover the costs with a check upon our departure.

After we had completed the third prostate operation and negotiations and rounds, we received the first true gift of the day.

When we checked on our prostate patient, we discovered one of our other patients toddling around asking for food, particularly candy. It was the three-year-old with pneumonia who had seemed so close to death that morning! His drooping drawers were almost at his knees, and it seemed that now his biggest trouble might be tripping over them. He was holding out his hand, saying, "Hunh! Hunh!" instead of grunting with each breath. There were lung sounds throughout all parts of his chest, and his fever was gone.

The crisis had tipped back over. As we watched him eat part of a banana, I thought, *So much for the triumph of surgical care as the highlight of this trip!* He was one more miracle to behold, and possibly the most precious.

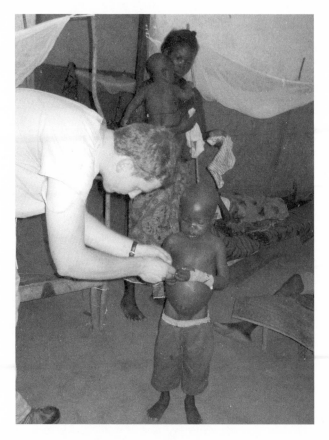

Pending pediatrician Josh shares a sweet treat with our miraculously recovered patient.
Now the biggest danger he faces seems to be losing his drawers.

Feeling uplifted, Josh, Dan, and I walked to the refugee camp near the Bangala-based Bible school. We had not gone very far when a man came to us in very polite greeting. He had a scar on his face from what seemed to have been a very significant injury some years before. He shook my hand very warmly and touched my hand to his head. I had already exhausted my Lingala greetings and social niceties and accepted his repeated "Blessings from God." We might have ended with this repetitive standoff had it not been for Les Harris, who had seen us coming in this direction and followed. Les also greeted the man in Pazande. The man insisted, however, and pointed to me repeatedly and explained something that made Les pause. "Do you not remember me? I certainly have never forgotten you!" Les translated. I did not understand until the man pulled up his shirt to reveal a scar where an abdominal incision had been made.

It all came back—more than twenty years whistled away and I was back in Assa looking over the crumpled form of a man who had just been dragged over to the theater.

"*Nyati!*"

Jean Marco and I had gone off hunting in the morning and had trekked over to a place he had named Mambassa (not to be confused with Mombassa, the Kenyan coastal port). We had crossed the tracks of a large group of dwarf forest Cape buffalo—*nyati*. They were among the meanest dudes of the rainforest bush. We had with us a few fellows who would help us porter the massive amount of meat back to the village in the event we should get lucky. We crossed over a dry streambed and tried to get in front of the herd; we could do so if we got lucky and they were meandering and not spooked. But instead, we blundered into the rear guard, and they thundered off, raising a cloud of dust, which was how we could tell how many and how far away they were and where they were heading.

We kept up the pursuit, going upwind and trying to intercept them if they circled back to where there was still water this late in the dry season. A big bull buffalo can use as much as forty liters of water a day, so the herd rarely strays too far from water. Part of the herd had circled, just as Jean Marco had predicted. I had crawled forward to view a group in the bush ahead of me, and

I focused on a big bull. He was staring toward me with his right shoulder visible and his head held high as he sniffed the air and swiveled his ears.

Jean Marco and I were alone with one of the porters, who was lagging behind us, while the others had been separated from us as the herd divided. The *nyati* were restless and stirring around, except for the bull, which stood still, as if fixated on me. Jean Marco was standing to the side, leaning into a small tree. Suddenly the .375 roared in my hands. The big bullet hit its mark exactly.

The bull had already figured out where we were and decided to close those hundred-plus meters with a double-time run. He had locked onto me despite my having tried to look a lot like the stunted tree into which I was leaning. He almost made it. He covered the first two-thirds of the distance in a graceful lumbering dash, and then crashed onto the hard earth just in front of me.

Jean Marco was grinning, since he knew I would not have been able to re-chamber in time. We took a few photos, one of which is in a frame in Derwood, next to the skull of the bull. We then began the long process of breaking down the quarters and packing back every last edible or usable bit. The porter who had remained close to us came up to see what had transpired and then left to collect the other porters. However, neither he nor the others returned. Jean Marco and I did what we could, collecting the tenderloin and "the book"—the unfolded compartments of the omogaster and rumen, a tripe-like delicacy for the Azande. It cannot be preserved by the usual drying and smoking, so is eaten right away.

After covering the partially butchered carcass with branches, we headed back to Assa, assuming we would meet the porters on the way.

But we did not. And when we got to the village, we discovered why. A small crowd of people, including the porters, were standing around the crumpled form of one man. The local clinic worker, Inikpio, was examining him. He had been gored through the abdomen and cut across the midface, which had opened the maxillary sinus and the underside of the right orbit. He had a facial fracture and his upper teeth were loose.

"What happened?" we asked.

The answer came back in a single word: *Nyati!*

The man was one of our porters. He had been with the group that had been cut off behind us. When Jean Marco and I had advanced on the herd and they had run off and circled back, the hunter and hunted swapped roles. They came back to have a look at what predator had been so audacious as to threaten them. The others in the group said that they had heard nothing and did not discover that this man was missing until the porter closer to us had come back to fetch them all. We had all been at risk, but he had been the unlucky one.

Inikpio and I got busy. I had a relationship with Merck at the time and the company had given me an investigational quantity of its new and potent antibiotic for surgical infections, imipenem (Primaxin). I had carried several vials of it with me to Assa, and if ever there was someone in desperate need of treatment for polymicrobial infection, it was this fellow!

I administered the first powerful doses of this third-generation antibiotic as Inikpio and I set out to treat him, almost as one would treat a war wound. We debrided the foreign bodies and the bluntly smashed tissue and bone from around his face and packed it open with gauze. We performed a spinal anesthetic and then opened the abdomen. We removed grass and dirt and debris, including some of his own clothing that had been rammed into his peritoneum (the abdominal cavity), and we debrided the tissue there as well. (Debridement is the removal of dead, infected, or severely damaged tissue and any foreign body or contamination to improve the healing of the healthy tissue around it.) Luckily, he had no colon penetration, so I did not think he needed a colostomy, and while the small bowel had been torn in two places, we fixed the tears. We used up all the sterile saline we had to wash out the belly and then put in gauze packs, which were slowly pulled out over the following days. Packing a wound with gauze and then removing it over time lets the healthy tissues granulate and heal naturally together; it's a better alternative than trying to suture together a lot of internal tissue in a way that may not be ideal for long-term repair.

What was most remarkable about this fellow's post-op recovery was that it was mostly unremarkable! He seemed to recover on schedule, which I am sure is more due to the debridement and open wound treatment than to his "first-in-class" antibiotic treatment, but he got that as well. However, he was still hospitalized when I left Assa. I had no one to ask about his follow-up, and I didn't return to Assa for seven years. I never knew how well he had recovered, or whether he had recovered at all. And here he stood, looking healthy and well, with no obvious disability. I said to Josh, who took our picture together, "This must be what heaven is like!" It was another gift, reminding me of the importance of the work we do here. Yet, of course, the plentiful blessings we receive from above are the primary source of any successful outcome.

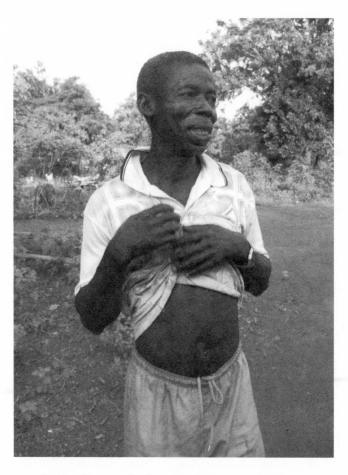

Fanigawa Jean, one of my hunting guides many years ago in Assa,
reveals the scars from a nyati, or Cape buffalo, attack.

While I was still marveling about this reunion, Les was startled in his own turn. We came upon a fellow sitting under a tree, in rapt attention to his trade. He was a knife maker.

Les explained that his name was Merci Andre, which sounded like what I eventually would say to him. Merci Andre was a fellow like all the others in the Zande territories, pursuing his livelihood, doing a little bit of farming and hunting and gathering. In 1978, as an adult, he'd noticed a numbness in his feet and gradually became unable to move the muscles of his lower limbs. It did not cause him severe illness, but of course became a major disability. At that time Les Harris had seen him. He realized that he had some kind of progressive transverse myelitis—an inflammation of the lower spinal cord. There hadn't been any distinct trauma or puncture of the spinal column, so it was possibly caused by a bacterial event.

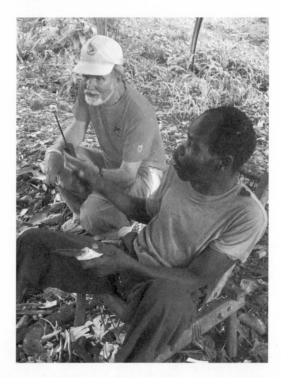

I study the tool that Merci Andre uses to create knives out of scrap metal and branches he can find for the handles. He has lost the use of his legs due to a spinal infection, but that has not reduced his contributions to the community.

As Merci Andre's disability hardened into a total loss of function of his lower extremities, Les had, in essence, written him off. *He's gone*, Les thought. *Life is tough enough around here without that kind of impairment.* "I would have given him a life expectancy of a year at most," Les told us. That was thirty years before.

Merci Andre had realized the same overwhelming odds he was up against. Having lost the use of his legs, he now crawled on his hands and dragged his knees, which were able to follow—he had enough control of hip flexion to pull himself along. Still, not a very life-enhancing set of abilities. But he did not beg. He did not curse God and die. He did not seek out the person who had cursed him, though it would've been a perfectly legitimate pursuit of justice among the Azande.

Instead, Merci Andre got busy. He was close to the ground, so he gathered up scrap metal and discarded parts. Soon, he had taught himself blacksmithing! He realized he could forge the scrap metal he found into new and more useful shapes. This entropy industry—taking castoff things and reducing them to make them more valuable—did not stop there. Over time he developed the skill of manufacturing what everyone here must have—a knife and other cutting implements.

When I saw Merci Andre seated under a tree with his useless lower extremities tucked under him, he was hard at work putting handles on two blades he had previously drawn out. He had made his own set of tools, which included an awl, and he was drilling holes in wooden handles with it. He said he especially liked the red duiker, a small bush antelope, as a source of the leather he tanned to make sheaths for his knives. He also enjoyed the crafting of a finished product, and was embarrassed that we had caught him in the cruder, earlier stages of production, since he decorates the handles and makes carvings and stainings of the accessory parts of the knife. Like makers of samurai swords in ancient Japan, he knows how many "foldovers" make a higher-quality blade of tempered steel. Merci Andre gathers this steel in many forms, including old automotive springs.

Josh, Dan, and I asked how much he required to make a knife for each of us, and he said he would have done a very special job if he had known how distinguished his buyers would be. A good knife would cost 500 CFAs (US $1), but a machete-sized blade would be 750 CFA. We were carrying no currency, but Les had a 1,000 CFA note and gave it to him for blades for Josh and Dan. Merci Andre gave them the blades he had just completed, apologizing for not having the time to decorate them fully. Now Dan and Josh had genuine souvenirs, courtesy of the self-taught skills of Merci Andre.

The knives were shown to the rest of the team that night at the long tutorial and wrap-up of the week at Zemio. The participants explained what they had learned and said how valuable the experience was. After we'd packed for departure at first light, we were all eager to get to bed; we needed to be up well before dawn for our convoy's launch. As I was heading to bed, I was interrupted by a *"Hodi, hodi"* at the door.

A man had arrived with a message from Merci Andre. The messenger apologized for him that he could not come this far dragging his lower half, but he did not want the "doctor who had come to visit to go away empty-handed." He knew that we were going to Obo for a week and that we would return to Zemio to leave the CAR. He would be working throughout the course of the week to make a knife for the doctor; the knife would be left with the doctor's bag in the Zemio station hangar. The messenger said that it was important that I recognize that this was a gift, and that no payment would be accepted. Merci Andre was delighted to do his part in thanking the doctor for his continuing care for the Azande, who have suffered so much. There was no reference made to Merci's own disability.

So I would be departing Zemio first thing on Sunday morning, again with gifts from the poor.

PART II

REACHING
THE POLE—OBO

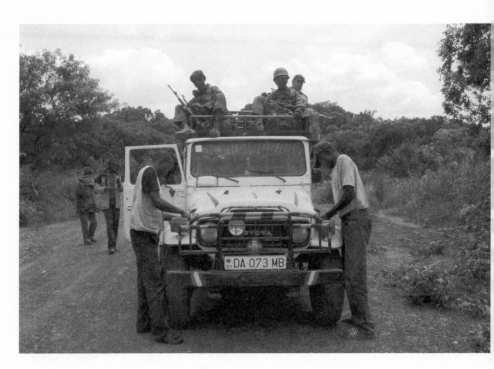

Our CAR security guard, up top on the metal rack in full battle dress uniform, with AK-47s.

Chapter Eight

The Medical Convoy

June 10, 2012, Zemio to Obo

IN THE ANNALS OF ADVENTURE TRAVEL, OUR "SAFARI" WOULD rank high on the list of most, well, adventurous.

Transecting a rainforest in the eastern CAR by road during the rainy season, especially when making the journey in two fragile trucks that have never encountered pavement in their long working lives, is exciting at best, nerve-wracking at worst. But we moved on with the blessing of Les and Mary Anne Harris. We had a ceremonial prayer at takeoff, and Les, who was concerned that I had given up my last dollar, presented me with a $100 bill, a contribution from his Florida church supporters. Mary Anne wished us Godspeed and sent us along with homemade buns and fresh peanut butter recently pounded in the mortars and mixed with honey. Some of the Assa Azande also showed up to see us off at the Zemio station, including Zapai, the caretaker of the station. He kindly didn't mention what we owed for our stay.

Some of our team was eager to ride in the open truck bed. I assured them that the adventure would quickly wear thin and that they would be better off inside the Land Cruiser. They reluctantly agreed, and even enclosed in the Land Cruiser the adventure *did* wear thin, for some even before we reached Zemio town. Joe, our videographer, did ride in the back of the truck, along with Celestine and Sacco, to shoot footage of our transit. We picked up our two CAR army guards from their barracks in Zemio, and they climbed into the back of the truck to be hoisted up to the rack on top. We stopped to pick up Ambroise as well. I had the chance to meet Madame Ambroise, who came to see him off, and Ambroise's father, the former sultan of Mboosa village. Ambroise's father was wearing a two-colored fur hat and looked regal, even though he had been displaced from his seat of power. We shook hands, and I congratulated him on his son's rise in status, which he accepted proudly. Through translation, he thanked me for my having helped enhance that potential.

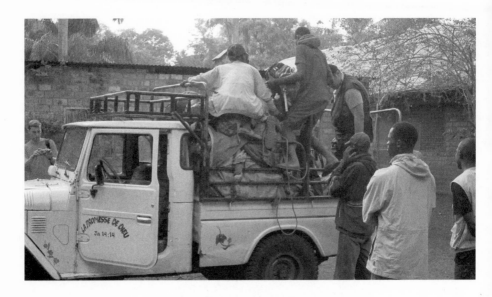

At 6:00 a.m., we load up the team and the gear at Zemio station for our adventurous trek through the rainy-season CAR.

I sat in the front seat of the Land Cruiser (which was marked with the decal of the Zemio medical clinic), wedged between Suleiman, the driver—who was also the Land Cruiser's mechanic—and Ambroise so we could make plans. Ambroise wanted to make several stops for medical diplomacy, which is so important in the region, and to show off the American professor of surgery who was assisting him in developing health care in the eastern CAR.

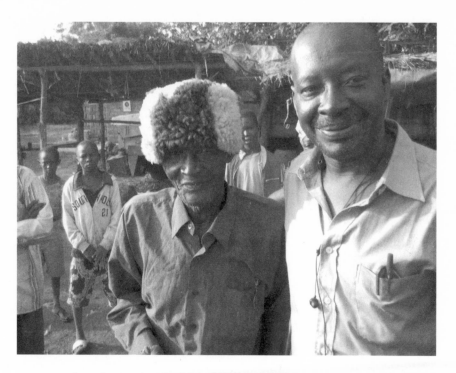

Father and son: Ambroise and the sultan of Mboosa, displaced now to Zemio town.

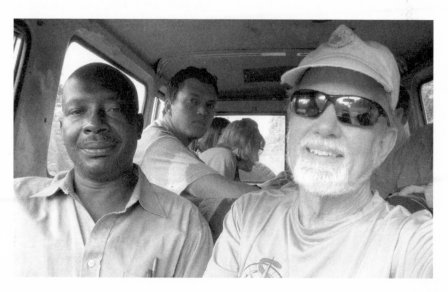

Bon voyage! I'm a bit cramped as we set off, in between Ambroise (left) and Suleiman, the driver.

We traveled along a primitive "road" that would take us through the villages of Mboosa, Jemma, and the wilds adjacent to Balanguie and Gouije, where, it had been reported, the wildlife had returned in good numbers since LRA activity had forced the poachers to evacuate. We would move on to Mboki and then Obo.

Ambroise projects at least three weeks for this road trip for the proposed mobile surgical mission of the future, operating four to six days in each village and carrying the convoy of equipment, including the generator and the operating microscope for cataracts. If we are to spend time in each village during a proposed mobile surgical mission, hauling a trailer that would serve as an OR along this route, we would need to plan for six weeks. I would have to create a "Team A" and "Team B," since few of the working team members could get six weeks off from their jobs back home. We would have to find a nexus where the outgoing Team A leaves and Team B is flown in. There is no air traffic here unless I charter it in and out. Access to transportation at the pole of inaccessibility, we had learned, is a very difficult thing; this place is on the way to nowhere!

Ambroise received a call from one of the local clinic workers in Obo (another miracle of modern communication), asking if we were indeed returning as I had promised in January. Apparently we had a glut of patients lined up for operations: fifty-nine goiters, forty-three hernias, nineteen gynecological or pelvic operations, and eighteen cataracts! There is no way we could operate on that many patients in Obo alone. Traditionally, there'd been a high fallout rate among patients who would have to travel long distances during the rainy season. We wouldn't know how many patients we would actually have to operate on until we arrived. From my years working in Africa, I knew we would have to remain *semper flexibilis*, or as the US Marine Corps jokes, "semper Gumby"—always flexible.

Our guides lovingly tended to the vehicles, and we stopped several times for on-road maintenance—to add oil and water, to replace lug nuts, and to ensure that the uneven terrain hadn't loosened any significant parts.

The road was a red ribbon of mud, two tracks cut through the jungle and small swaths of grassland. Because the rainy season had come later than usual this year, the roads were better than I anticipated. I'd feared they might resemble the tropical mountain-slope mud troughs we had slogged our way through on recent missions to Haiti and Burma. In fact, the conditions here were nearly ideal—wet surfaces with occasional rutted passages and puddles. Going through big, muddy puddles along a slick roadway may constitute a hazard, but it is far more pleasant for the following vehicle, particularly for those riding in the back of a pickup truck. In the dry season the passengers of the second vehicle of the convoy would be enveloped in red clouds of road dust for hours on end.

Smaller villages were strung out along the road between the larger villages we would stop in, but a large amount of our transit was through long stretches of jungle that looked to be impenetrable beyond the roadside margin. One guard riding on the pickup was almost swiped off by the overhanging vegetation, but he was saved by his uniform, particularly the clip pouches for the AK-47 ammo magazines, which snagged on the roof rack.

My principal interaction with the armed escort included taking photos of their precarious perch atop the cab of the truck, like the emblematic bulldog on a Mack Truck, and swapping mango sections with them; they used their bayonets to peel green mangoes whenever we stopped for a "mechanical break" or to go back and pick up something that fell off the truck.

We often had francolins or guinea fowl on the run in front of the vehicle, unaccustomed to traffic. They would take off in front of us at odd angles that would not get them out of the truck's path. We came close to scoring a few fowl for lunch. It wasn't surprising that they used the road for their own path; we met only two vehicles along the red road. The first was a big truck with the words "Union City, New Jersey" on the side. Standing passengers— heads held low to avoid being pummeled by branches and vines, knees bent to absorb the jostling—held tightly to the railing surrounding the bed of the truck. The second was another Toyota Land Cruiser that passed us slowly while we were waiting on the side of the road for our truck to retrieve a bag that had fallen off.

I snapped a photo of the truck and a very nervous fellow stopped the vehicle, jumped out, and asked why I had taken his picture. He was working for a humanitarian NGO and assessing hunger in this war-torn region. Ambroise spoke with him in French, matching his animated speech and letting him know we were every bit the humanitarians he was. It turned out he was worried about the LRA. He would have freaked out if he'd first met our truck with the armed CAR soldiers.

We could have showed him the big and imposing folder with the official-looking travel permits and all the stamps and signatures on it, which authorized us to take a "short cruise through the central African rainforest." The rubber stamps were the same as those of the agents at Zemio who punched our passports, which of course we had with us, certifying that we had purchased the mandatory $200 visas for this luxurious tour of the CAR countryside.

We were perhaps the least injurious and most beneficial of any of the foreign invaders in the region.

The larger villages we stopped in looked quite similar to Zemio, as they were mission stations, too. And as in Zemio, indigenous pastors, Bible school teachers, station managers, and CAR staff carry on the work of the original missionaries of AIM.

We made the mandatory visit to Mboosa. I shook hands with the chief, who knew Andre the Dentiste and Inikpio, my Assa trainees in the Congo, from whom he had learned about me. We stopped many other times along the way for diplomatic greetings if there were any subchief who needed a hand shaken. One of these had had a pterygium—a benign growth of the conjunctiva, the outer pink covering of the white of the eye—operated on by Ambroise, and another pointed at me and at his thyroidectomy scar! That is what I like—follow-up hut calls at the pole of inaccessibility.

At every stop, we saw proof of all the locals who, it seemed, had voted for Barack Obama. At least two or three people in each village were sporting

T-shirts that displayed the likeness or logo of the president. Several women had T-shirts that said "Obama Girl." There were also several Canadian maple leaf emblems. But the favorite T-shirt of the trip was "Disco Still Sucks," worn by our own Isaiah.

We crossed the Kerre River, the border between the Zemio and Obo subprefectures, on a fixed pontoon ferry. The rains had not yet been heavy enough to require that the ferry be pulled across the river; a series of ramps on each side of the cable-anchored steel drums floating in the middle of the river were enough to get us across. From the riverbank, an explosion of colorful butterflies erupted into the air. Along the road, wherever there was moisture, such as big puddles or even dung piles, red, yellow, and white butterflies hung out with those of their own color but would rise up in waves of Technicolor brilliance as we passed.

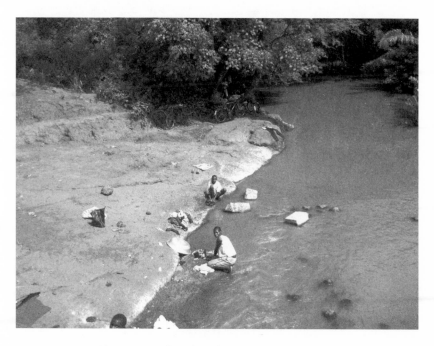

The Kerre River, boundary of Zemio and Mboki provinces.

As we entered Mboki, one of the largest villages between Zemio and Obo—if not *the* largest—a change occurred, startling in its abruptness. The town of Mboki looked like Am Timan in Chad, overwhelmed by the presence of the Mbororo (a subgroup of the Fulani tribe) instead of the Zande and Bantu peoples we had been passing. The majority of the men wore the white, flowing robes and rolled turbans of the Arabic-speaking desert tribesmen; the women were colorful, with gold hoop earrings and brightly colored gowns. How they walk out of the muddy roads and appear like spotless dazzling flowers I do not understand. When the Harrises were at Mboki, it was a predominantly Bantu, Zande, and Christian community with a church and Bible school. Now it seemed to have become an Arabic-speaking Muslim village of nomadic pastoralists.

The home of the Mbororo has always been in the western grasslands of Africa along the Sahel, and I recognized them from my early travels in Nigeria, a half continent away. Their presence is a product of the desertification of the Sahel, or the spreading of the Sahara. As they followed the Hajj routes on their pilgrimages to Mecca, they discovered the lush green areas of rainforest to the east.

This area of the CAR is a game reserve, specifically a noncattle area, from which only the Azande are entitled to extract resources as part of their hunter-gatherer lifestyle. The Azande need a very pristine wilderness in which to survive. As soon as the Mbororo bring in their cattle, the game vanishes because the indigenous animals don't want to or can't compete with large, dense herds for grass, water, and other resources. They can't live in an area once it's been foraged out by the cattle herds.

If the Mbororo don't move on, and if the CAR doesn't exert its right to protect these lands, the Zande way of life could become severely threatened. And aside from obvious cultural clashes between the Mbororo and the Azande, tensions are also high because the Mbororo have been suspected of supporting the LRA. In reality, it seems that Joseph Kony just uses the Mbororo to disguise his movements and to get access to both cattle and women. They are likely as victimized as any of the other people in the LRA's path.

There is a hospital at the outskirts of town where Médecins Sans Frontières/Doctors Without Borders runs a good midwifery service. They flagged us down, and a couple of the MSF staff recognized me from my January trip

to Zemio. There was a short, young woman who looked Mbororo with scoliosis and rickets and a full-term pregnancy. The woman had been picked up
by an emergency vehicle for transfer to the midwife. The emergency vehicle?
A motorbike. Consider the comfort level here: a woman in early labor being
bounced over muddy roads for miles on the back of a motorbike. Given her
condition, she would certainly need a C-section, and the midwife told me
they were capable of doing one. Our help wasn't needed, and so we moved on.

Our rather long and very deliberate diplomatic break at Mboki was like
falling into a family reunion. We got drinks in recycled Fanta bottles and met
other Soungouzas, including Ambroise's brother. Isaiah also introduced us
to two of his brothers; it didn't seem like such a big deal to see three of the
siblings in one place, but then Isaiah reported that he had fifteen brothers!
When I asked him how many sisters he had, he added as an afterthought, "I
may have as many as five." To be startled by such information requires the
mindset of the Western world. Here polygamy makes for unusual family sizes
and age proximity of half-siblings.

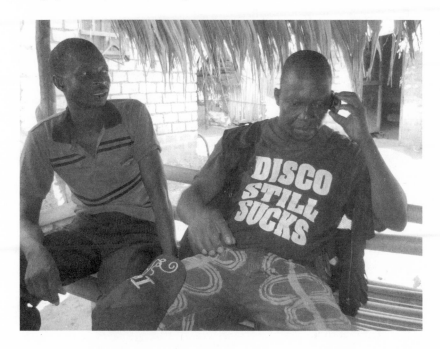

Isaiah (right) wears his ludicrous "formal" T-shirt as he sits with one of his fifteen brothers.

Ambroise's brother's wife had died of a postpartum hemorrhage about four months before. The cute, four-month-old baby girl was being cared for by her aunt, Ambroise's sister. Orphans here are often absorbed by the extended family without so much as a discussion. Who else would care for them? The baby was passed from team member to team member while her father and aunt asked if I could furnish baby formula, since the aunt is not able to nurse the child. All children are breast-fed here, and wet-nursing is not a cultural custom. At Derwood, I had formula stocked, but it was too heavy and too much of an investment to bring along. It's not a sustainable practice to carry food into the field. The baby looked to be in good condition, though, so whatever nutrient source they were giving her seemed to be working. In a couple of months they wouldn't have to worry about it.

I was introduced to the bishop—or chief pastor—of the Mboki church, Maku-Bagudekia. He spoke English well, had lived in Bangui and Uganda (hence his facility with English), and even gave me his Yahoo! email address. He has a pharmacy in Mboki that supports him, in addition to his work for the church. The bishop called himself "best friend of Ambroise" and, accordingly, had a request. He had a family member who was a student at Isiro in the DRC and he wanted him to come for a visit to Mboki. He asked if I could please call up Jon Hildebrandt, since I was chartering aircraft to fly all over central Africa, and ask him to make a special flight to Isiro to pick up this student and deliver him here when he comes to retrieve us from Obo in a week. There was either much naïveté or the bishop was shooting the moon, figuring it couldn't hurt to ask. We were tooling around three different nation-states, with passports and visas in hand, right? A quick hop over to Isiro with a Cessna 208 Caravan that burns a barrel and a half of jet fuel per hour to pick up a single person would cost as much as the exorbitant investment we were making just to get our team in and out. He was asking for a favor equivalent to donating a used Land Cruiser. I explained that I had no phone and no way to reach Jon, but that he would be contacting us by the end of the week and we would see which route he was taking to retrieve us, and I left it at that.

I walked over to the compound of the church. Inside, there were a number of the deacons counting up proceeds from the collections and making arrangements, in the form of small piles of Central African francs, for how much should go to which worthy causes in their community. I was introduced to many of them and then shook hands with the pastor. After we greeted each other, I was told he had been summoned from his sickbed, to which he had retreated with bad diarrhea.

Unfortunately, I hadn't packed any Purell hand sanitizer.

After completing our diplomatic rounds through Mboki, we got our convoy started again over the small fords and bridges to the east of the town. Along the road in the Zemio subprefecture, we had seen encampments of Congolese refugees set up in virgin forest, supported by the outside world, namely UNHCR and NGOs. The encampments were covered with plastic sheeting (distributed by UNHCR) over thatching. The inhabitants all share in the poverty and despair of their displacement, although some of the camps appear to be better organized than the villages they replaced, since they are aligned on the terrain in an orderly system. In fact, they look much like the Congolese village structures around Zemio, which were planned and instituted before UNHCR was even aware that the Congolese had been displaced and moved into the area.

Past the small rivers outside of Mboki, though, we encountered the abandoned refugee settlements of the South Sudanese. They had come into the CAR in two major waves. In 1968, during the Sudanese Civil War, when Sharia law was imposed, foreigners were expelled, and bombing began in South Sudan, the South Sudan refugees were resettled here in UNHCR camps and didn't return home until 1974. The second major wave came in 1989, when the south rebelled under John Garang, giving rise to the "Lost Boys" who fled from their cattle camps. These refugee camps overflowed again under UNHCR, until the South Sudanese returned in 2006, under the terms of the Comprehensive Peace Agreement. That agreement mandated the referendum of January 9, 2011, which resulted in the secession and creation of the new state of the Republic of South Sudan on July 9 that same year.

The jungle eventually, and sometimes rapidly, reclaims modifications to the environment and any signs of human habitation. The green jungle around us had once been an instant town of refugees, but the regenerative power of the rainforest was recovering and erasing the signs. I could see second-growth areas with stumps of giant hardwoods, but otherwise it looked like the virgin rainforest through which we had come.

We stopped in the small village of Kadjiou, and I watched some women in the process of mutual grooming. In sociology or cultural anthropology, one learns a lot about how grooming practices are linked to social cohesion, but these women were clearly deriving a practical benefit, too. A couple of women had wiry hair standing out like they had been victims of a failed electrocution. A third woman had gone to work on their hair with a small rake and was pulling out large hanks.

A pile of the shed hair was stacked next to the woman in a tangle. A fourth woman came forward to harvest this hair and began to spin it with a suspended stone that pulled it out into a long strand. I didn't stay long enough to follow the next step, but I was curious. Perhaps the hair would be turned into a wig or woven into a "hair shirt" to keep the donor of the hair warm!

We reached the Boho River and crossed over another pontoon bridge that becomes a floating ferry in the later rainy season. As we parted another curtain of red and then white butterflies swarming over the stagnant waters of the Boho River, we entered Obo.

We emerged from the butterfly heaven of the rainforest and pulled into the Obo mission station in midafternoon, driving along a course of road that seemed familiar to me. I realized it was the path shown in a YouTube video posted a few years ago about the African pole of inaccessibility and areas of LRA activity. In the middle of the road was a makeshift turnstile created by a pike set across the track. The gendarmerie on post was busy slicing mangoes, and the men took their time getting up to let us through. When they did, one of them recognized me and shouted, "Aho! You are back, as you said you would be!" He stamped and initialed our "internal visa" and we waited for the truck to come along with our supplies.

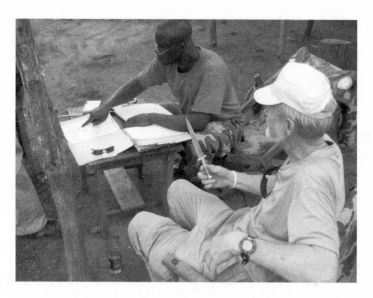

Checking in at the "office" required meeting with three sets of armed forces—the CAR army, the UPDF, and US Special Forces.

Once we were all through, we drove to the improvised OR to unload our supplies. A mud and wattle building with several rooms would serve once again as our consultation area. Adjacent to it was a building that would house the post-op patients—more patients than had ever been seen in Obo, even during its heyday of expatriate mission staffing. A third building was used as a delivery room, but it would become our two-table operating theater, as it had been in January, and storage place for the instruments. In January, it had contained three operating lights—an incandescent light bulb, a truck headlight, and a Castle overhead OR lamp, none of which worked. We had done most of our operations with each of us wearing a headlamp. This time, we had brought better lighting with us, two photoflood lights. The ends of the tables drop down to make deliveries easier, so we would have to prop them up. Outside was a large, nonfunctioning steam autoclave, now displaced by our kerosene stove and pressure cooker. Before the instruments were wrapped in cloth to be "cooked," they would be scrubbed and set out on a platform that seemed tailor-made for this purpose. Closer examination revealed that it had once been an ironing board in the mission station.

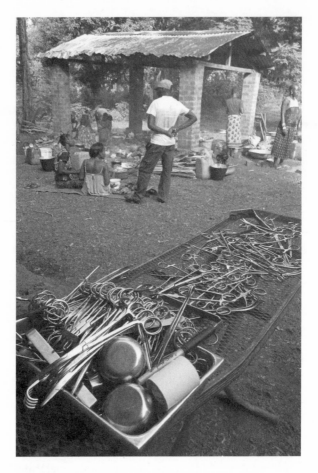

What was once an ironing board is now an instrument-drying rack.

Ambroise suggested we wait until tomorrow to set up our instruments and OR and to visit the AFRICOM battalion in Obo. I suggested instead that we go immediately to the battalion, introduce ourselves, and try to set up tonight so that we could begin a full-court press first thing in the morning. AFRICOM is camped near the African Union troops, namely the UPDF, near the old CAR army base, which is now mostly in ruins. We delivered our CAR army guards there and then approached the AFRICOM camp.

Despite the fact that they stand out, most would not guess that the ripped young guys who wear Hawaiian shirts that barely conceal the 9mm Glocks at their waists and who drive around in new Ford pickup trucks are US Army Special Forces. They are only offering "logistical support" to the African Union and the UPDF, which had the bad habit of surrounding Joseph Kony and his entourage and then somehow never closing the ring. Kony kept slipping through. The suspicion was that since the UPDF knew that if they actually captured him, the $1.5-million-a-day gravy train sponsored by the United States would be over, they didn't try as hard as they might to actually do so. Under increasing pressure from Congress, AFRICOM took the reluctant step of assigning US Army Special Forces to keep an eye on the UPDF-led efforts to see that they really do what they say they are here to do.

Prior to the March 2013 coup in the CAR, the Séléka coalition had been taking control of villages in the eastern part of the country. They were chasing down anyone who had arms and ammunition. The US Army Special Forces in Obo had enough firepower to make a coup a nonevent, but there were 120 fellows sitting behind concertina wire just itching for the rebels to try to steal their ammo. They're not supposed to lay a finger on Joseph Kony and they would just hunker down inside their encampment if the rebel forces had moved into Obo. But they're also waiting for some action. The rebels were smart enough to realize that if they pulled on that tail, they would receive a big kick.

We stopped at the rolls of concertina and razor wire and I gave the guards my name and passport, asking if I could enter. They looked under the vehicle to inspect it, but said it could not come in and neither could the cameras. I agreed to that, and sent in my card. Very shortly, out came the team! The master sergeant and chief operations officer, Chris, was out immediately and brought with him Captain Paul. They had heard all about me from Captain Craig and his team, whom I had enlisted to help when we were here in January and who had pulled out a month before. The enthusiasm of their greeting was why I wanted to come directly here. We had the last team starting IVs and carrying patients in and out of the theater, and we let them in on some of our tutorials. I had grander plans for this group, and I wanted to plant the seeds right away.

Chris and Paul explained that they had been told only that "Dr. G. and his team would come and do amazing things" and that the medics "have got to try to be part of it." So they invited us into the chow tent, where I introduced the entire team, including Ambroise and Isaiah, and met the two medics with the battalion, Dys and John. Dys had done an Internet search on me before arriving here two weeks ago and had shared the information he gathered on my background. He'd seen that I am a runner, as he is. Sadly, neither he nor I had done any running since arriving in Africa, and would be unlikely to do so given the OR schedule I was predicting.

Dys and John had trained with a lot of good equipment, but it was mostly done on simulators and on each other. Their experience with us would go a bit beyond that! We toured their med tent, which was air-conditioned, a thrill we could not let ourselves get used to. They had an abundance of everything, including a Polar monitor—a self-contained unit that functioned as a blood pressure and heart rate monitor, a pulse oximeter, and an EKG device—to replace ours, which had become a weight for holding down the curtains. They had powerful gooseneck operating lights—a real bonus—in addition to lots of surgical gloves, some sutures and supplies, and a few drugs, including narcotics that would make our general anesthesia easier with less dependence on ketamine.

They promised to come over that night as we set up the OR and bring along some stuff we might borrow. Chris told me he would send over a truckload of bottled water and cases of MREs (Meals Ready to Eat). I promised them they would be doing everything I had taught the team, including spinal anesthetics and suturing up operative wounds for closures. They could scarcely believe it—a training program in the real world with real patients and a real teacher!

The evening found us working alongside the US Army Special Forces team to finish up the OR setup so we could hit the ground running tomorrow at 7:00 a.m. I learned that John and Dys were leaving on Thursday to go to

Djibouti in order to handle the paperwork of re-upping for another six years. I got serious with Dys, counseling him with the former US Army motto: "Be all you can be." I encouraged him to consider something more than being an army medic and to learn about the Uniformed Services University of the Health Sciences, where he could go through medical school and then work in the medical corps. I hoped that the one quote I gave him from Thomas Carlyle, the Scottish philosopher, gave him pause: "The tragedy of human life is not so much what men suffer, but rather what they miss."

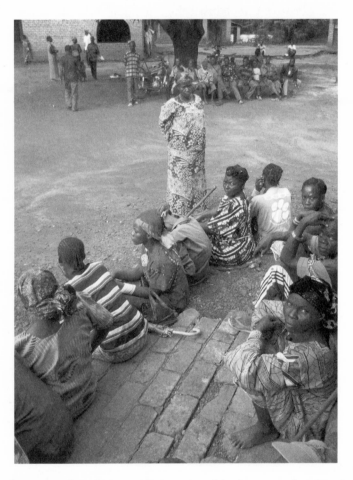

My "waiting room" outside the consultation room and the pharmacy we brought with us.

Chapter Nine

Reunion on a Hectic Opening Day

June 11, 2012, Obo

Five o'clock a.m. The rhythmic drumming of the wake-up call resounded to scatter the usual cacophony of dawn birdsong, which had followed the forlorn wail of feral dogs. Through the night, we'd heard the hippos down near the river and a few hyenas, as I'd warned the team we would.

We had now visited the poignant relics of multiple mission stations, built in the heyday of "trek missionaries." These pioneers would scout out unreached areas, determining the local population, identifying the water sources and access routes, and looking for a bluff hilltop on which to build a mission station. Eventually these stations would be turned over to the local churches or seized by local groups. But today, many have come to resemble ancient ruins, in at least their architectural features, which are still somewhat out of place in the terrain. The Obo station, like the Zemio station, is well situated, framed with bougainvillea and frangipani, but still seems haunting, like the sign of a civilization that has come and gone.

This would be a big day—we would see a massive number of patients and one very special one. Hundreds of patients lined up outside our consultation room. Apparently, thanks to the good road conditions, the scheduled patient fallout rate wasn't very high.

We tried to get an early start to the operating series by stacking up patients for each of our two operating tables. I had fit in a few consultations after our arrival the day before, and I immediately began to see more people, in between running over to take each of the team members, including medics John and Dys, through spinal anesthetics. These two fellows jumped with glee into the deep end of the pool as additions to our swim team.

We filled two tables and rotated teams between them. At each table we had at least one medical student (Dan or Josh), one CFA, one of the special forces team, and Isaiah or Ambroise to perform the operation, depending on whether or not I was needed. Ambroise was the chief medical officer, Isaiah performed a running series of hernia operations with help from various assistants, and I was delegated the role of chief credentialed advisor and instructor. One table was stocked with women with pelvic or abdominal masses, like large uterine myomas or ovarian cysts that required spinal anesthetics. The other table was filled with a succession of men with hernias, both inguinal and otherwise, as well as one man with a large hydrocele. Throughout the operating day we added three laparotomies and at least three goiters from the consultations I continued to do.

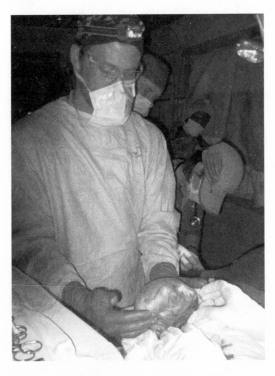

Dan and Josh admire bilateral hydroceles.

Captain Richard—a captain who was out when we arrived last night but who remembered me from my previous visit—and Sergeant Chris came over with a group of curious troops, including the special weapons officers and others who could scarcely believe that their medics were operating in a small mission outpatient clinic. I walked them through the process. The group included three men who wanted to talk hunting with me, as a few of the locals were going to take them out on Saturday and show them some areas where there is still game—a day after I am gone! I told them I wanted a bongo and that they should save one for me.

The US Army Special Forces team will likely view this as a pinnacle experience of their stay in the CAR, primarily because it's unlike every other day of sitting and waiting, interrupted by drilling, eating, and pumping iron to shed the excess weight gained from the instantly accessible MREs.

I started the day hungry because I had passed on dinner the night before. Isaiah had brought along a special treat from home, already cooked. But it had spent a long day in transit without refrigeration. The special treat was hard to identify in the kerosene lantern light, so we asked what it was. It was described as a "little animal." When the quartered pieces of the "little animal" were passed to me in a bowl, I looked down to find large incisor teeth bared up at me. It resembled a miniature beaver. Dan didn't have the advantage of light and hadn't made such an observation. When he crunched down on his first bite, he realized that he was crushing the skull in his teeth, the skull of an animal that seemed equipped to bite him back! We made jokes about ROUSs—rodents of unusual size. Only Bruce might have appreciated this treat less than Dan—he had gotten the tail end of the same creature.

The US Army Special Forces came to our rescue. We had *no* chance of being finished with cases during daylight hours, and our exhausted team would be going back at dark more interested in sleep than trying to find something to eat. The special forces showed up in a truck to deliver a "few goodies." There were about six cartons of MREs, an abundance of bottled water, and a "Café-to-Go" instant coffee brewing kit. So in the middle of the day as we rotated our cases off the table and were finishing our consultations, we brought out the team and a few of the local folk for their first high-calorie treats—courtesy of your tax dollars.

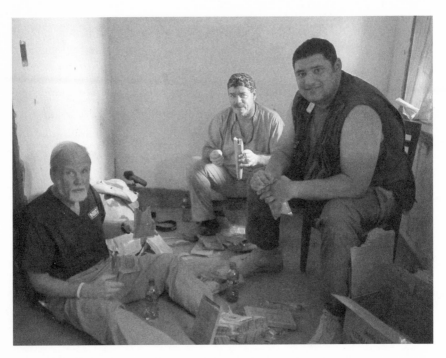

We chow down at midday on the US Special Forces' rations of MREs.

Contrary to what I have often said, "MRE" does stand for "Meals Ready to Eat," *not* "Meals Rejected by Ethiopians." They come packed with amazing exothermic chemical toaster ovens, activated by mixing water with the packaged salts in a plastic bag. They're available in a large variety of flavors and are superb if you understand that they are designed to be eaten when no other food is available and when you may only get to eat once a day. The American Heart Association would probably not recommend them, since they are high in calories (packing in over 2,500) and are often high in fat. They even come with matches if you carry your own cigarettes, and there was a time when they came with Lucky Strikes. (Except for a few of the CAR soldiers, I have not seen people smoking. Only the uniformed men seem to have the disposable income for the habit.)

I had a "Chicken Pesto" MRE for lunch, and others, like Leenta and Claudia, shared a few different flavors, diversifying their first MRE experience. Many of the patients were walking around that afternoon with little packets that said "Chocolate Peanut Butter." I had eaten MREs in Louisiana at the Hurricane Katrina rescue operation, so the thrill for me was a bit lost. I wouldn't want to subsist on them; however, if I were fighting in an advanced position at wartime, I would appreciate the once-per-day feedings. The advertising logos on the overpackaged, hard-to-tear envelopes say "This food is a 'Force Multiplier,'" or "This is a high performance food for the field"—as if anyone consuming these foods in emergency situations needs encouragement to choose them over the alternatives.

In addition to Chiclets and Skittles, there were a few good items, such as "Cranberries, Osmotic," which I presume is the army's way of saying "dried cranberries." But the favorite item is a package of what should be called "animal crackers" but is labeled "Patriotic Cookies." The small cookies are pressed into a "USA" logo, the American flag, or the Liberty Bell. I am sure the guys in the field need the cookies to keep them gung ho.

The best part of the delivery, though, was the cases of bottled water. On nearly every trip, particularly to the hottest climates, a major portion of each day is devoted to procuring and sterilizing enough water to keep us going. When we had arrived in Zemio in January, we had already spent weeks in other countries in the region and I was so dehydrated that I wasn't peeing more than once a day, despite drinking whatever water I could find. Now, we fearlessly guzzled water. Still, despite drinking multiple liters over the coming days, we would rarely pee. We go into the OR wearing rather heavy-gauge, high-quality OR scrubs that certainly don't help with the dehydration. I realized I needed to ask Jerry Kekos, who had donated these high-quality scrubs through NIFA, to find cheap scrubs to allow me to get through the days here without sweltering!

Of all the clothing I packed, probably the most useful pieces are the LA

Marathon shirts. They are made of fabric that wicks away perspiration in distance running.

We never have to worry about trashing the environment with an excess of empty water bottles here. They can hardly hit the ground before they are eagerly claimed as home appliances by the locals. It reminded me of Rwanda, where the kids would see us coming and start yelling "*Aga jupa!*" which means "small vessel or container." They know that wherever white people and tourists go, water bottles are dropped along behind them, and those bottles beat calabashes and gourds for carrying liquids. We had rules: We would toss bottles to kids, but no one wearing shoes, and if the kids had only shorts or wore minimal clothes that looked very threadbare, they got more.

Despite the bits of modernity offered by the US camp, our reality is still very low tech. The Honda generator runs for about forty-five minutes on a full tank of a couple of liters of kerosene. No one thinks to buy ten liters of fuel to have standing by when the tank empties and the generator sputters out. When that happens, we struggle on through the dark, grabbing for available headlamps, and a fellow on a bike is sent to fetch fuel—just enough to fill the small tank. We get the generator going again, and forty-five minutes later, the process is repeated.

In central Africa, you go to market every day and buy two small bread rolls. Why? Because if you bought a dozen, everyone would know and they would just come and get them. After all, you couldn't possibly eat them all yourself. This is another reason that people rarely buy cell phone SIM cards with more than fifteen minutes. If you had more than fifteen, somebody would borrow your phone and make a long call. And here, they sell fuel by the Coke bottle, because if you have more than that, anyone is entitled to come and siphon it. Life is lived day by day. The less stuff you have, the lower your profile as a target of predation.

Our low-tech approach applies to everything, not just lighting. We have early ambulation and post-op care stylized to a fault. Following a big and difficult procedure, the patient is assisted to a sitting position, mopped of all the blood, helped down from the table (without a footstool), and assisted in dressing him- or herself. With this minimal help, one of us, sometimes me, walks the patient out of the theater to the door, which is held closed by a trash bag that has been pushed against it. As soon as we emerge into the dazzling light from the darkness of our OR cave, we encounter a group of people, many of whom are seated on piles of green leaves they have torn off the nearest bush to offer some padding against the hard laterite.

As we make our way out of the OR in slow motion, supporting the stiff strides of the patient, one or more people—relatives—separate themselves from the group and join us, helping the patient to the "recovery room." If no relative pops up, a bandaged patient will usually come forward to help. In the recovery room, the patient will lie on the planks of a mattress-less wooden cot. Then patient and helpers will clasp their hands over mine and murmur, "*Merci mengi.*"

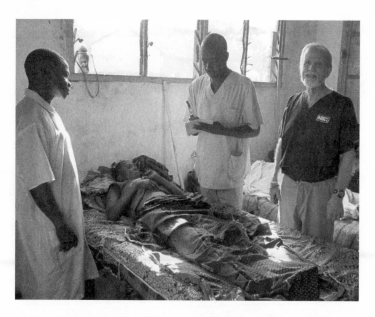

Celestine, Ambroise, and I make rounds on the post-op patient who was Dys's first lumbar-puncture spinal anesthetic.

I then return to start the cycle all over again.

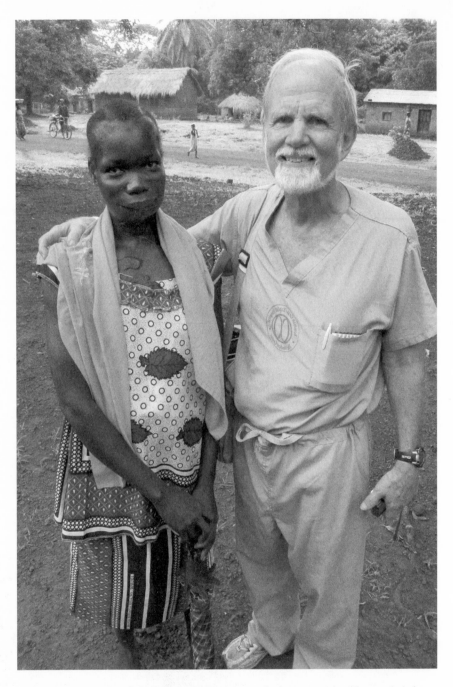

Flore comes to greet us. It's the first time I've seen her since the dramatic events of five months before. After extensive surgical excision and reconstruction, she is now on HAART drugs for HIV.

Amid the rush and the scramble of the day, we had an amazing high point. It came early and it helped give us inspiration. Our premier patient was Flore! She was all smiles, at least to the degree she could manage with her bone and tissue graft stapled around her reconstructed mandible. She was not reluctant to show her face, as she had been in January; however, she still carried her scarf in one hand, gracefully veiling her face, presumably so as not to frighten small children with the still-healing incisions of her extensive facial resection and reconstruction. She saw me from where she waited under a tree with her brother, Blaise, and ran to meet me. She had come a long way through this experience; she was no longer the shy young lady I had first met as she hugged me now. I introduced Flore to the team members who had not met her before but who knew her from her dramatic pre-operative photos. It was gratifying to see them all in a state of wonder, as if they were seeing her raised from the dead.

We headed into the consultation room and I called Dan and Ambroise over. Flore could manage a smile and even eat in a normal way. She had put on some weight, because she could eat better and because she was on the HAART drug combination offered by Merlin, a British NGO that provides health care and drugs to remote areas. If she continues to follow the regimen rigorously, she might have a nearly normal life expectancy, and at least be present while her five children are growing up. She reported that she was happy to be back home in Obo with all her family, especially her children.

She had been relieved of her malignancy, the most immediate threat to her life. But the surgical treatment of her malignant disease had also uncovered her potentially lethal viral infection. Left unattended, either would've been a death sentence, in short order. We had taken a worthwhile chance with the operation, and I would do it again if I were presented with the situation today, even knowing of her HIV status.

We started up my laptop and I showed her the photo of her pre-op appearance, taken in the same room less than six months before. Her eyes grew wide, as if she could hardly remember what the cancer was like in its unsightly ferocity! Her sister and mother came in from outside, and I turned the screen toward them. They had looks of shock and horror, as though they'd forgotten, too. I turned back to Flore and saw tears rolling down her face. It was the only time I ever saw her cry.

Flore was ready for follow-up. She had a small staple in her suture line, which I removed with the assistance of John from special forces. She will continue to be diligently monitored; the local medics will look for any evidence of recurrence of the resected tumor and will control her HIV status, closely monitoring her lifelong regular schedule of HAART drugs. I wrote a note with a post-op photo to the Kijabe Hospital that I would email much later, when I could find Internet access, to let them know of her progress and her reunion with family here.

In Pazande, she offered her thanks into our tape recorder. I had hoped to have our reunion captured on film—Flore is central to our return to Obo—but Joe was not to be found. Apparently he had gone to town in one of the vehicles. So I scheduled another interview with Flore and her family for the next morning.

Watching them leave, Dan said, "Now I can say it. I was dead set against this. I thought it was a waste of money. Now look at her."

_ı́⁛⁚ꞥ_

By the end of the day, the members of the team were shaking their heads. They had thought they were functioning wide open and full out at Zemio. Now they saw the light. We had accomplished a dozen cases and done untold consultations. Some had observed their first-ever hernias or assisted with their first hysterectomies. AFRICOM personnel were seeing and doing things they had never imagined; they may have entered hoping to start a few IVs, but they did much more.

Their captain urged us to come over to take advantage of a newly rigged "shower," which sounded too good to be true, having been in a sauna all day. We took them up on their offer, maybe only for the sake of the ride over, which offered a cool nighttime breeze.

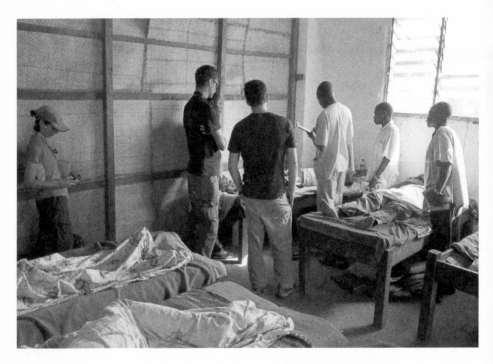

I turn post-op rounds with Claudia, Dys, Dan, Ambroise, Celestine, and Sacco into tutorials, as we have already overfilled the infirmary.

CHAPTER TEN

TWO TABLES, THIRTY-EIGHT CASES

June 12–13, 2012, Obo

WE KEPT THE OPERATING GOING FULL TILT FOR DAYS. WE WOULD do at least fifteen operations on our second day. We had to work faster, particularly as we were offered cases wholesale in batches. A local nurse in charge of the community center came over with a carefully outlined list of eleven cases, each of which had a diagnosis of some pre-op condition labeled with the patient's name. He was proposing adding one full day of operations to our schedule. And we would need to see each in consultations beforehand, to verify the diagnosis and determine whether there were any further complications to be anticipated.

I had everyone doing everything, and by the end of day three we had about thirty post-op patients overflowing the beds and spilling onto the floor between them. We numbered them as I had at Takum Christian Hospital in Nigeria back in 1968: bed one, "bed" one and a half, bed two, "bed" two and a half, and so on.

Our two soon-to-be medical students, Dan and Josh, had become expert independent operators. They had graduated from practicing suture knots on shoelaces during the Ethiopian Airlines flight to Africa to doing every manner of closure, specializing in bilateral hernias, assisting each other while standing on opposite sides of a patient. They were doing a really good job. Bruce had tied knots before but never as a first assistant or while working deep in the pelvis suturing the broad ligaments. Claudia had done some suturing when she was with me in South Sudan last year, but she had become a regular fascia-on-up closure expert, as had Leenta. Claudia would take another big step in the coming days, too. Everyone stayed busy doing something they'd never done before—and in some cases never dreamed they might. Some even graduated to "teaching" it.

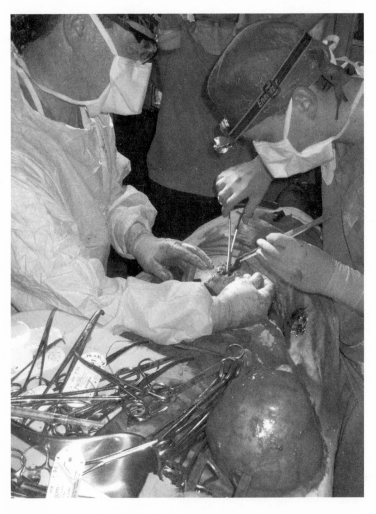

Josh VanderWall, incoming freshman medical student, carrying out skin closure with the assistance of soon-to-be-certified CFA Bruce Visniski. Note the specimen on the Mayo stand.

Despite the flood of operative candidates, we had been conservative in our patient selection; we were not there to stamp out disease in Obo or the CAR, but to take the most difficult cases that were still fixable and diagnose the simpler ones that may be done by the indigenous team with the supplies we would leave behind. They were cautious in the new techniques they learned, clearly understanding that they must apply them with careful judgment, which they borrowed from me while I was still present. None have overreached.

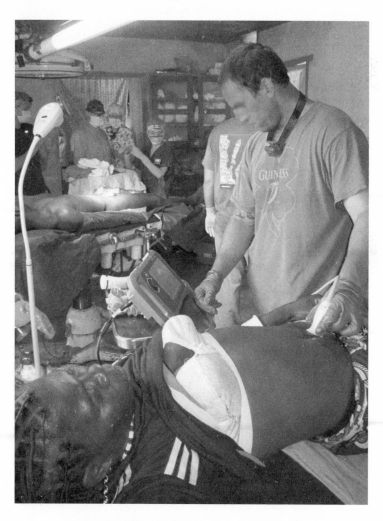

The first use of the SonoSite, used here to rule this woman in for medical management of pelvic inflammatory disease.

We booked a score of hernias for the following week, and the Zemio team, having already done cataract operations there, would start those operations here on our final day and then continue in earnest on the Monday following our departure. We also invited the AFRICOM medics to participate with Ambroise and Isaiah. By then, the medics should be confident in these two men, who are cautious and careful and deliver good results. My hope was that they would come and learn from them—and also carry along some additional supplies, as we were running through our consumables at such a rate that only the largesse of the US military would be able to keep us supplied.

The military had already helped us immeasurably. We were able to approach the cases for the day with more appropriate technology, rather than the entirely low-tech approach we'd been taking. The AFRICOM team raided its supplies to supplement ours. We had use of not only good monitoring units but also a brand new SonoSite, which costs about the same as a Land Rover and is one of the most useful pieces of imaging equipment for a medical mission. I even extended the technology further by getting the Interson probe, which can be hooked to a laptop so that the results can be displayed there. We used it to scan women with possible abdominal or pelvic masses and to image problems in the abdomen or other parts of the body. Given or loaned the kinds of equipment and supplies we were more used to, we could be even more efficient—just when we needed that greater efficiency.

We had had four women in consultation with gynecological problems; either they had never started menstruating or had stopped prematurely, or they had never been pregnant or were unable to become pregnant again. One was especially interesting; she seemed to be hyperthyroid, with agitation, tachycardia, and sleeplessness. But she had no goiter and didn't have enough iodine intake from the surrounding environment to become thyrotoxic. What we found was an abdominal mass, left of center and mobile. She could have been one of those rare ovarian teratoma patents who become thyrotoxic from an ovarian source. We would have to operate to see the nature of this semisolid mass. What we knew from the ultrasound was that it was not a cyst;

it was ideal to get the pre-op picture sonographically confirmed and to see the nature of the lesion.

After our first flurry of ultrasounds on OR table one, we had an interruption. There was turmoil in the large and colorful crowd outside. A trauma patient was already in the "emergency room," a bench in the clinic where a few of our personnel stood next to a sign that advertised the clinic. The man had been brought in with head trauma resulting from a stabbing during a fight that had occurred in town the night before. Apparently quite a few of the people involved were outside the theater. The faithful and hardworking Isaiah was inside suturing up the scalp laceration. It was long but superficial, and mainly caused by the blunt force of the blow. Curiously, I had just emphasized the underappreciated blunt component of penetrating trauma in the tutorial the night before.

During a brief respite, I met with a former Ugandan Catholic missionary who now works with Cooperazione Internazionale (COOPI), an Italian NGO that fights poverty and assists populations hard-hit by emergencies. He was interested in our work, but was puzzled by my affiliation and was trying to determine what organization I was with. He assumed that with a name like Mission to Heal, we were some big organization that had plenty of funders to pay bills and salaries. I tried to convince him that I am simply a low-drag, high-mobility operator with a small group of volunteers. I don't need to report to central headquarters or seek permission from a board of directors. I go where the need is greatest. On that day, it was Obo.

After a few more complicated hernia cases, goiters became the operation du jour on our second and third days in the theater. Goiter patients require an injectable systemic anesthetic agent beyond local infiltration of anesthetic in the skin and soft tissues. Since we now had access to Versed, morphine, and a few other agents from the AFRICOM stock, we would not have to risk the hallucinations and possible psychotic breaks of a ketamine OD.

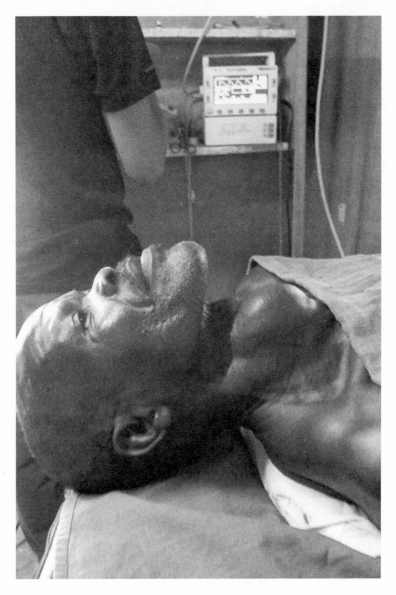

A stoic Zande fellow with goiter awaits atropine, ketamine,
and Versed—our general anesthetic equivalent.

In these operations, we pushed everyone to his or her maximum point of competence. Our usual method was for me to free up a goiter from all the significant attachments and dissect it away from any danger points, such as the important recurrent laryngeal nerves and blood vessels. I controlled the goiters on a final pedicle, or point of connection to the surrounding tissue, with two clamps. The scrub nurse or assistant would then excise the big gland, so that he or she is the one to do the climactic (for them) part of the operation, the part where the patient and the disease part company.

Many of those assisting got the chance to excise a goiter, and Isaiah did his first-ever thyroidectomy, and then still more after. Dys assisted Isaiah by managing the IV anesthesia in a balance of medications observed carefully with the loaned monitoring system. Claudia had a major first. I had gone through the prep of a goiter and the patient was now draped and ready; I advised her to proceed with the skin incision. "You are kidding, aren't you?" she asked. She was hesitant, as are all new surgical interns, and did not cut deeply and swiftly enough, a common issue for first-time "cutters."

The final goiter operation of the second day and many of those on the third day were "foolers." These patients didn't have very large visible goiters, but they did have significant airway or food passage obstruction. But what we discovered once we had opened them up was that, like any good iceberg, the majority of it was out of sight, hiding in the chest, below the manubrium of the sternum. This is the upper part of the sternum in the middle of the chest; it attaches at the top to the two clavicles and below that to the cartilage of the ribs. It makes a good hiding place for some very large goiters. We pulled these large masses from the chest up through the cervical "collar incision."

They were dumbbell shaped, with a significant indentation in the mid-portion that we might have mistaken for the isthmus of the thyroid, a mistake that we actually made at first. The deep groove was caused by the clavicle, which the goiter had grown around. The symptomatic piece, in terms of obstruction of the esophagus, was the larger one in the chest. In a couple of cases, the goiter in the neck was sizeable but nowhere near the size of the actual mass inside the chest. If we had been less attentive, we might have excised the large mass in the neck, dividing it at the isthmus of the dumbbell, and left the more symptomatic piece in the chest.

The army medics, John and Dys, watched with fascination, muttering, "This is unbelievable!"

_..,ıı:::ı..._

The morning of our third day was an emotional one. I patrolled around the house before the others had gotten up and then went to the church in the center of the mission station. A couple of our team members went to the local Catholic church while I walked to the indigenous Zande church. When I arrived, only the pastor was there, sitting at the front with a Bible and his glasses. Four men and one woman eventually appeared and the service began. In the brick structure, open above the walls and below the eaves, the sound was quite impressive. The attendees sang in harmony that became an eight-part echo of four voices. I walked around the church and photographed the handmade architecture, including the brick flying buttresses. This church will stand over time.

As I returned from this very brief interlude before breakfast, I was approached by Flore's brother, Blaise. With only a word between us, I realized we were to miss another opportunity. I had scheduled them for a video interview on the first day; however, our videographer was often wandering about doing something else, and he missed it. Flore had returned later in the day, and he missed that as well. So I asked her and her family to come for an interview with Ambroise. We wanted to share it to thank the people who were involved and who supported her in this very unusual and expensive undertaking. But again our videographer, who knew of the planned visit, was away.

The whole family had gathered at the house, so I set up both of my small cameras and made a homemade video. Ambroise described how we had met them and his stay with them for a month in Kijabe. Each family member expressed his or her gratitude, preceding thanks with the statement, "We have nothing to give you!" They thanked God for making our encounter possible.

I ran into the house and brought out a print of the picture I had taken of Flore when I first met her. Her mother looked at the picture, and Flore held it up next to her, as a dramatic before and after. Her mother shook her head, clicked her tongue, and cried. Once again, she faced the certain death that had been present on her daughter's face.

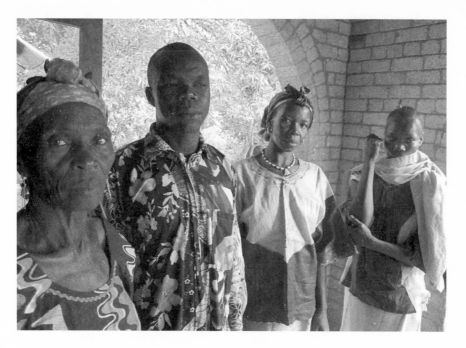

Flore's mother; her brother, Blaise; her sister, who cared for her five children in her month of absence; and Flore herself, now back in Obo.

The OR was a sauna, with no air circulation. While we were grateful for the gooseneck lamps loaned to us by the US Army Special Forces medics, they were intensely hot, particularly because we positioned them right over the operating field, which meant right next to the operator's ear. We had run out of size seven-and-a-half sterile gloves, so I made do with size sevens, which were too tight. As we ran out of more and more disposable items, I hoped we might take it up with our army volunteers. We would need their help in order for the local team to continue after our departure; we were burning through supplies fast.

I helped Josh do a difficult spinal that turned out to be a highly successful blockade. And thank goodness, too, because it turned out to be a life-saving operation. The patient had bilateral ovarian tumors, which looked to be cancerous. The cancer had clearly started on one ovary and metastasized to the other. But there were no signs of metastasis in the omentum or peritoneum. If we truly did get it all, we may have prolonged the woman's life by untold years. She wouldn't have access to anticancer medications. Although we had seen some tamoxifen here, which I had left for a breast cancer I had encountered in January, there was no consistent supply line, so this operation would be her only shot at controlling the cancer.

As we were working, Isaiah was struggling to keep a patient on the table. The man had a hernia and was sitting up, wild eyed, and looked ready to jump down and run for it. But Isaiah is superb at comforting and calming patients. He got the man to lie down and accept a local anesthetic and then kept him calm throughout a successful hernia repair. In each operation, the people look up in wonder, and sometimes fear, as their insides are on display. It isn't surprising that it is unnerving for some. Consider what the response to this high-volume "disassembly line" might be in a first-world environment.

During one of the quick consults between operations, I saw a young boy who had a large sebaceous cyst—a sac beneath the skin that is filled with keratin and sebaceous secretion, a fatty, semisolid substance that is produced by sebaceous glands in the skin—behind his right ear. The cyst was pushing his ear forward. Draining a sebaceous cyst is quite simple, so I told Josh, as he was downing an MRE, that I had found a case for him to operate on and took him through it after our hypercaloric lunch. I helped as the young boy jumped up onto the OR table and, without a whimper, submitted to a local anesthetic, incision, drainage, packing with an iodoform wick (gauze placed into the wound with a small piece emerging to allow for further drainage), and dressing—all done with his cooperation.

But not every patient we saw presented such a clear-cut opportunity to help. In the clinic I saw a woman who had a large mass in her abdomen, very clearly defined with an edge that crossed over from left to right, went down to the iliac crest (the edge of the pelvis that creates the prominence of our hips), and dipped down into the pelvis. It was easy to determine what she had: tropical splenomegaly syndrome. The cause? The same thing that causes so many problems here—malaria. When the body is exposed to malaria infection again and again over years, the immune system becomes overstimulated and the spleen becomes very enlarged. The huge spleen is what I was palpating in this woman's abdomen.

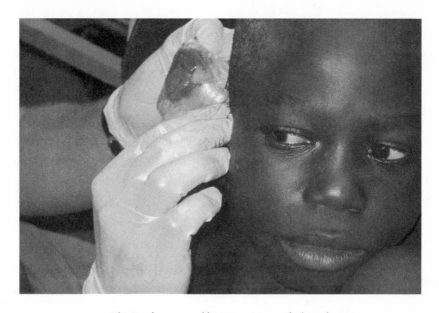

This Zande ten-year-old is just curious, not frightened.
He accepts the excision of a sebaceous cyst behind his ear as a rite of passage.

I brought her over to see the other members of the team so they would have an opportunity to identify this problem and diagnose it. The answer did not come from the medics without coaching, but to Dan, it was apparent right away. He had seen an earlier clinical exam of a patient when he was with me in Am Timan, Chad. The highest-profile patient there was a man with the same diagnosis. Dan had felt the enlarged spleen and witnessed me doing a splenectomy using the autotransfusion technique of returning a large amount of sequestered blood that was trapped in the enlarged spleen back into circulation.

Why not attempt to do the same here? Not in Obo. Hypersplenism can cause blood-clotting difficulties. That complication made it likely that we would need blood transfusions. Without refrigeration and donor screening for HIV and hepatitis, there was no way we could use any blood there. I could

not run the risk of excessive hemorrhage without access to blood or labora-
tory support to confirm platelet counts that would tell us whether she had
good clotting potential. This was one of the many judgment calls we have to
make; an operation that *can* be done must be judged against the factors that
are warning us that it should *not* be. An elective operation that one might "get
away with" puts the patient, not the doctor, at risk when we fail. We don't do
this work to look good through our "heroic" successes. A splenectomy would
require a weeklong inpatient stay, following an extensive operation with venti-
lator support and a stay in the ICU, which would require many other support
services. Despite the fact that our day began with a celebration of the success
of just such an endeavor, we would treat this patient with antimalarials and
the Pneumovax vaccine. The spleen, when functioning normally, protects us
against "encapsulated" organisms, like pneumococcus and meningococcus;
thus, the patient was at risk of developing lethal septicemia if exposed to such
organisms. With these medications, she could continue on, although with an
increased risk of rupturing her spleen if she experienced any trauma.

In the future, maybe the required operation would be possible here, but it
would have to wait.

At the end of our third day, we got out early enough to take off our wringing-
wet scrubs and go to the battalion for a "luxurious" warm-water shower, as we
had on Monday night. Afterward, we would join our medics, Captain Paul,
Sergeant Chris, and others for a pig roast. Paul and Chris met us at the gate
and helped us enter, for the first time without extensive frisking by the UPDF.
They even allowed our driver, Suleiman, to drive the vehicle around the base.
The whole team contributed to our operation, and I wanted to be sure that
Ambroise, Isaiah, Sacco, and Celestine, and even our drivers, were properly
represented.

Our dinner got off to an unplanned start. The pig that had been the
planned entrée was now in an aluminum foil pouch piled high with the
embers of a wood fire. The pig's demise was unusual. It had been standing

under the brush to which it was tethered, panting in the heat. Hondo, the cook and special construction help, came over to the hog and, figuring it was hot, took some cold water and poured it over the pig. The pig expressed its gratitude by falling over dead.

So the pig was dressed out a bit earlier than planned and then put on the coals a bit too directly. When we arrived, the medics rather sheepishly pulled back the foil to show that the pig had been virtually incinerated. Dys and John started peeling away the charred, black eschar to salvage a bit of the pork. Meanwhile, a goat was slaughtered and put on the fire.

We spent a little time making a very brief circle around the town of Obo to see the village center, which was run down with heavily rutted clay roads. We saw a number of *majlis*, or groups of Arabic men in long white robes, sitting in a circle on a rug, discussing the problems of the day, and drinking Arabic coffee. Then we returned to the base.

Exhausted, we were silent and drowsy in the dark during the cooking process. Chris told us about his wife and thirteen-year-old son in Colorado and how desperately eager he is to see his boy go to college, something Chris had not done himself. The structure of his life was the special forces, and he had been separated from his wife for most of their marriage and his son for most of his thirteen years. He will be going home after retirement in three years. He discussed the grand adventures he has had with the special forces, serving two tours in Iraq, one in Afghanistan, and now his second in Africa. We talked about the advantages and disadvantages of the life in khaki, and I told him I was in conversation with Dys about the Uniformed Services University of the Health Sciences.

When the thermometer showed that our goat was finally ready, we came through the mess tent to help ourselves, piling meat onto tin plates along with helpings of rice and "pulled pork" salvaged from the pig. We had packaged peaches and pound cake for dessert. We spent a good portion of the dinner in silence. But people began popping in (they had heard there was a special non-MRE meal being served for guests), including one fellow named Scott who was with the State Department and was supposed to be checking in on all LRA issues in this part of the world, and a fellow named Ken, the military liaison officer who is based in Bangui and had not been this far east before. And we saw Mark Pearson. I hadn't been sure if we would see him on this trip, despite the fact that he had been researching whether we might get transport from Zemio to Obo with the UPDF. When we saw him here in January, he had been functioning as an interpreter and translator for the US Army Special Forces, but he plays many roles here and in Bangui.

Mark and Ken were both interested in what I had been doing and were eager to learn more. I introduced them to Ambroise (whom Mark had already met) and Isaiah and encouraged them to help these two after we leave and in the future, when I might be back in the action with them. We spent a long time comparing notes, and everyone in the US Army Special Forces agreed that ours was the single biggest boost to the medical program for the medics as well as a big positive for their tour to date. All were grateful to be of help. We struck a very positive note in military/medical/political diplomacy. A long evening of waiting for dinner to get done, and not overdone, resulted in a good series of liaisons that might bring support for the work here.

After this, we would be working without either of the medics or some of the equipment the special forces had shared with us. But we had worked without them before. Aren't we supposed to be used to deprivation in materiel and personnel? As I retreated from the army's hot-water shower tent, I thought, *How easily one can adapt to relatively minor luxuries!*

At the end of our third day we had about fifty post-op patients—amazingly, all without any complications—overflowing our facilities. Encampments with cooking fires surrounded the buildings as the caregiving families supplied food and lower-level nursing care to the patients. It was gratifying to hear the chorus of *umhs* as we passed through; we saluted them with a wave or some other indication that we were glad to help. Every move we make is followed by a hundred pairs of eyes, and as a consequence, we try to be smiling, waving, and kind, regardless of the hurry we might be in to get on to the next activity.

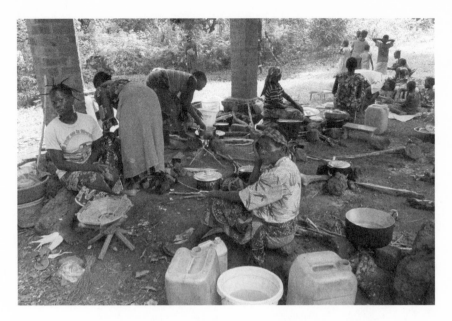

The caregivers and family retinue of our expanding inpatient population (which now fills not only all the infirmary beds but also the floor between the beds).

I am also cautious. The women in the camps navigate in the dark, barefoot, with a baby on their back and a load of firewood and a bidon of water balanced atop their heads. They will look around at me as I approach slowly in the night, as I try to avoid stumbling over the hard laterite or a termite mound and spilling anything I am carrying. The immediate response from anyone observing such an accident is "Oh, sorry, sorry," as though they are the direct cause of our clumsiness. They are often just as gracious and concerned about each other, carrying in food for the unattended patients.

After all, they speak the same language, so why would they not help?

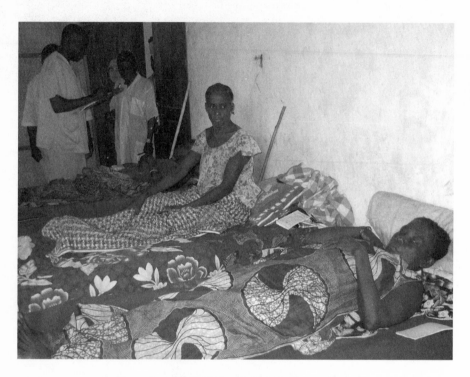

*In Obo, early ambulation is the rule. Note the absence of bedpans
and the presence of a sturdy walking stick.*

CHAPTER ELEVEN

LAST DAYS AMONG "ORPHANS"

June 14–15, 2012, Obo

AS WE MADE ROUNDS ON OUR FOURTH OPERATING MORNING, THE skies were dark with clouds and the wind was cooling. After the heat and high humidity of the preceding days, it almost felt like light-jacket weather. But it also meant that big-time heavy rains were on the way, and when they came, both our pre-op patients and those waiting for consultations might scatter for cover, leaving us with empty OR tables. We'd lose precious time as we searched for them.

Joe the videographer was with us this time, and he captured on film all the people doing well as we made rounds. The buildings were overflowing, with women in one large room on bed frames and men scattered about in other miscellaneous places. Some of the places where patients had come to rest looked like the Black Hole of Calcutta; no light came into the buildings even at midday, and people navigated by feeling their way along the walls, trying not to step on others.

As we entered the women's ward, Claudia asked me if the patients had been out of bed. I asked her if she saw any bedpans. No, she said. I pointed to the large walking sticks propped up next to the beds. Here, as in Zemio, early ambulation is the rule. When a woman is exhausted from a bloody delivery process, the midwives admonish her, saying, "Look at the mess you made—you clean this place up!" It might seem heartless, but it produces better post-op results.

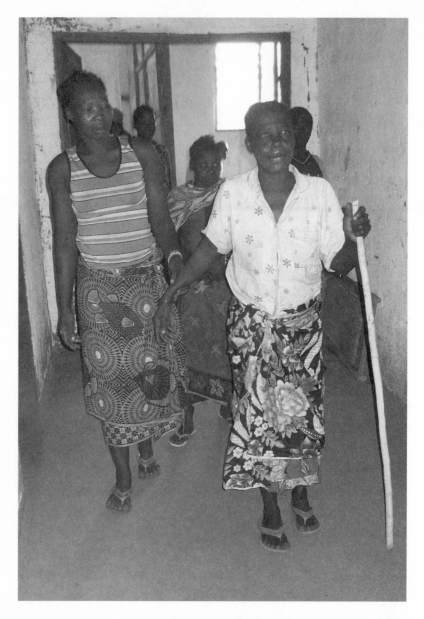

Assisted early post-op ambulation.

On our rounds, no one had a fever, all drains were pulled, all dressings were dry. Since rain was about ready to pour, we had to scramble quickly to the OR building to see the pre-ops for the day.

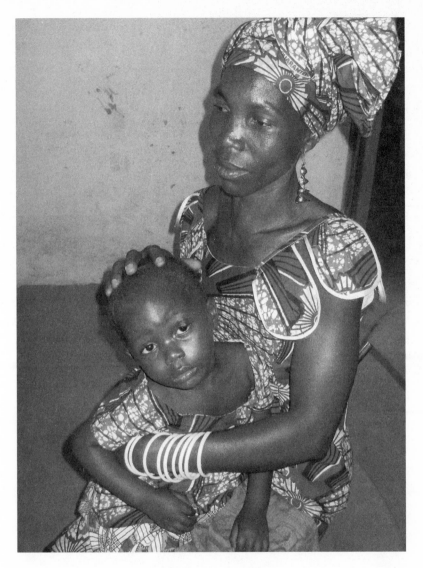

A Zande mother and daughter.

We added an additional operating day, staying on until Saturday morning instead of leaving Friday morning. The AIM AIR plane was initially reported to be arriving on Friday, but then we heard, through a delayed message on Ambroise's phone, that it would not be coming to Obo first, but to Zemio. It would be a more efficient use of our time, anyway, though we'd have little downtime anywhere, including in Entebbe. We would have to jam our flights, both charter and commercial, almost end to end. But it would decrease the hotel rates in Entebbe, which are more expensive than our rate here. It would also decrease our Ugandan sightseeing time, though, which was too bad, but we would still be able to insert a brief bit of tourism.

Under the assumption that we would be leaving relatively early on Friday, we had been focusing on the more difficult cases and postponing some simpler ones, including cataract operations and refractions (measuring for glasses, should any ever be available), since only one assistant was needed for those procedures. But now that we had another full day, we would work on filling up that OR time. Most of the cataract patients had been told to return on Monday, but we scheduled some of the new consults for our final day, when I would be there to observe. But Ambroise and Isaiah would be the primary ophthalmologic surgeons.

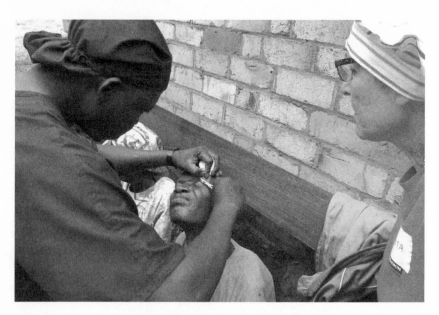

Leenta observes Isaiah at work clipping eyelashes—secondary prevention for trachoma, an infectious disease of the eye.

I wanted to encourage them to become increasingly independent. As I introduced them to the various government and military liaisons the night before, I made it clear that Ambroise and Isaiah were the primary operators of this mission and knew what could be done and where to be most effective. This was all very true. During consultations, we saw a woman with a left inguinal hernia who had had a prior laparotomy for a uterine myoma. Later, I asked Ambroise if he had done the laparotomy. He said he could not remember. I asked, "What do you have to remember? Since no one else is operating from here to Bangui and since she has an abdominal surgical scar, it's not a big intuitive leap to think that you did her previous operation!"

When the heavy tropical rainstorm hit, it scattered the families sitting outside. Ambroise was being interviewed by Joe, giving answers in a mixture of Pazande, French, and English. The downpour and the interview ended the assembly-line efficiency of the OR, and we still had not gone to see the group of eleven patients the local nurse had asked us to see—so we had two operating tables standing open and empty. As nature abhors a vacuum, I quickly walked the woman with the direct left inguinal hernia over to get her started.

I then proceeded to a fellow waiting in the mud-churning rain. He was a classic desert herder with a head wrap of coarse burlap the same color as his flowing robe, a robe he probably never changed even once as he traveled across the desert. I asked if he was Mbororo, to which he vigorously assented. We cast about in French and Arabic as I tried to determine his language. He said *Fulfulde*, the Fulani word for their language. When I said that the Hausa were from west Africa and that he might know that language, he brightened up, which wasn't surprising. The Hausa and Fulani are often considered collectively because they are ethnically related and because their stories have been intertwined by history. I knew a few words in Hausa from my work in Nigeria. I pointed to Ambroise and to me and said we were *likita*, or doctors. Now he knew what we were talking about!

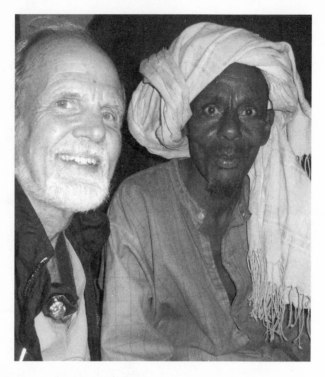

My Fulani friend, a nomadic cattle herder who came in for a "no waiting" hernia operation.

We found that he had a hernia, and I quickly scooped him up out of the consultations and brought him to the OR through the rain, since we could operate on him under local anesthetic. After a brief recovery he would be on his way again, a nomad still pushing east from western Africa, following his cattle and their need for water and grazing.

During a brief break after the rain, as I was trying to charge my laptop and my camera batteries, a fellow came up to me and opened a burlap bag to reveal two tusks. I immediately recognized them as belonging to a giant forest hog—a *zigba*. He wanted to sell them, and I agreed to buy them for 2,000 CFAs. I talked with him about what other trophies he had and where he had obtained them. It turned out that there was an area close by that held game. I suggested that since we had a vehicle and fuel and were now working with an extra day in Obo, we should go and look! But I received the same answer I always do: *"La prochaine fois"*—the next time. I have been promised wonderful hunts, especially in the area between Jemma and Bagunine. Since the LRA came through and drove out the people there, there has been no sustenance poaching for over three years, and the animal stock has proliferated to the point that we could find bongo or other species of the CAR rainforest in greater abundance than ever before.

I asked what weapon he had, and he replied, "Zero. Zero." Without a lot of translation help, it seemed that his was a homemade shotgun, probably made from outdoor plumbing left exposed. Ambroise said he would make inquiries for me as to how I might carry in (and out) a weapon and would try to find out whether there is a permit for transport of trophies. I continue to hope to be once again on the hunt in central Africa, after being far too long excluded from it.

Between ongoing operations and a few consultations, we grabbed an MRE lunch. I was almost bowled over by very eager cleaners, who competed for the honor of tidying up after us. There was a lot of mud tracked in by the heavy rainstorm. The special tools the locals use are homemade and interesting. One is a broom, which is a group of rushes wound together by the cuff of a disposed surgical glove. Nothing seems to go to waste here. Gathering the rushes requires the women to bend over fully from the waist, flexed at the hips, going about their business stooped like this for extended periods of time. It made me hurt just looking at them.

But they are not as eager to get at the muddy floor as they are to find their way through the big boxes of gifts—the cartons of MREs and bottled water dropped off by the US Army Special Forces. Just the leftovers from our hyper-caloric lunch could feed a whole village for weeks! I cannot imagine what the food would do to a family used to pounding their greens in a mortar and pestle and then adding the mandatory *ugali*, as it would be called on the east African coast—a paste made from cassava flour and water. If one of the indigenous people has eaten his fill of other foods and is then asked whether he has eaten, he will answer no unless he has had this heavy, starchy staple. It is like rice in many other parts of the world. Would they feel the same after eating heavy-duty MREs?

The goat feast planned for the evening could have the same effect on me.

In the evening, we experienced a second emergence of termites! At nearly every fence post and flagpole and around any stick or landing place, terrestrial termites emerged precisely six hours after the thunderstorms, after sundown. Oriented to the moon, they tried to mate and fulfill their biologic destiny, and then crashed to earth in a mad dash to get back underground before myriad creatures emerged to gorge on them.

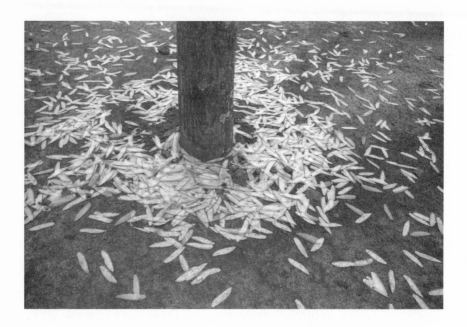

The ground around every pole is littered with cast-off termite wings.

The people of Obo were primed for this hatch, as they'd been in Zemio. The lavish outpouring of termites was scooped up with great joy by all ages, but especially children. The termites' arrival spawned another series of biological events, though. Out came other creatures that were also prepared for the event. About four hours after the hatch came the chorus of toads. The amphibians emerged like large blobs and hopped slowly around, lapping up the insects. Mounds of termites formed under any source of illumination, such as kerosene lanterns. Some of the toads were lucky enough to sit atop one of these mounds, devouring the perches on which they sat.

Another four hours later, the next tier of predators arrived—not a pleasant event for anybody with a snake phobia, like Bruce. The serpents emerged to stuff themselves with the toads. We did not venture out to view the third wave. We had already had too many close encounters of the reptilian kind for a few of the team. For Bruce's sake, we limited our serious snake sightings to Zemio.

Eventually, after all the gorging was complete, our tropical world came up with a contented burp. As dawn approached, the animals commenced their drowsy shuffle to find cover for a long daylight snooze.

_____ 🐚 _____

The evening's festivities—another goat roast and staff reception—might have been a comical sight to watch from a distance. To be a part of it was a bit of a challenge.

The speeches were translated into several languages, as a swarm of long-winged termites buzzed about, landing on the faces of the speakers or even dropping into their mouths. This was nothing new to the locals, and they didn't react like the Westerners, who do not ordinarily go through after-dinner speeches amid a major termite hatch.

Each speech given by one of the locals was begun with greetings to the family of the team members, thanking them for allowing us to be here, and pleas for God's blessings upon us. They asked that neither we nor God forget their impoverished people. The chief pastor said that it was obvious that God had blessed our efforts since we had treated so many patients and since all are doing well, without a single death among them. He did not add that Ambroise and Isaiah would do more operations during the following week. Then the speeches turned to lists of requests for help from those who had once supported the people here but who now had abandoned these orphans of the world. *Orphans* was their word, not mine.

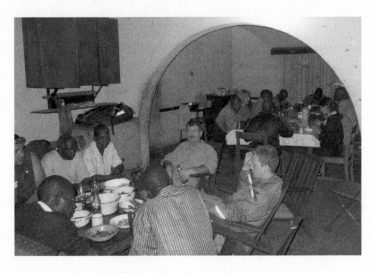

At dinner, hosted by the Obo staff during the heavy termite hatch.

In conversations throughout the evening, I was told multiple times that the people of Obo had been abandoned, neglected, and left alone to fend for themselves in circumstances not of their own making, completely isolated from those who had once cared for and supported them. They are now cut off from such support and from communications with those who had been here before. They used to use a shortwave radio, which they called the *phonee*, to communicate with the other missions, but the radio no longer works. In fact, operating the radio had been one of the prime jobs in the village and provided an opportunity to learn English. A man who had once been the phonee operator for the mission approached me almost in tears. "Now what am I supposed to do?" he asked.

When I heard them call themselves orphans, I asked, "How can you be orphans when we have the same Father?" They said that all the Azande were very poor and had nothing to give us. I pointed out that the title of my last book, *Gifts from the Poor*, was selected because they *had* enriched and encouraged us so much. They repeated over and over that we must return often (oblivious to the expense and logistics of bringing a medical mission to the pole of inaccessibility) and stay longer.

One of the pleas was for us to return during the dry season, when we could see many more patients, since people would be out in the *shambas*—gardens—during the rainy season, trying to cultivate what little keeps them alive. It made me wonder how many more patients we could possibly treat than the record number we had just seen. They did not seem to realize that we were operating this week on the large number of residual patients we hadn't been able to operate on when we were here in January—during the dry season.

They also seemed envious that Zemio not only gets more visitors—of course, both times we have gone to Zemio, we also went to Obo—but also has five assistants, when they have zero here (discounting John, who pulls teeth). They had heard that we had both Emmanuel and Sacco there as trainees, and they noted that there are no assistants in training here in Obo. They wanted such programs so that all could learn.

Unlike the refugees from Assa around Zemio, many did not know of my longstanding relationships with the Azande in the DRC, in South Sudan, and in the CAR, and thought that maybe I was an explorer just discovering their tribe for the first time. They did not know that I had promised to help them in a much better way—something more than "helping" them become dependent on come-and-go foreigners again. I told them of the hoped-for next trip, during which we would support Obo's own indigenous health-care workers. I said we might include Rafai, Jemma, and Mboki, as well as the Mboosa and Zemio and Obo regions, but only to train their own health-care workers to treat the people resident there, and not only because I was following refugees from the Congo, with whom I have had over a generation of relationships.

"I'm here to make sure you're taken care of well by the people you already have in place here. We're going to try to enhance their skills, and this will make you more independent," I told them.

The response I heard, twice, was "We don't want to be independent; we want to depend on you." I actually had to ask for it to be repeated because I wasn't sure I had heard the translation correctly. They seem to want neocolonialism; even if they might be treated as second-class citizens in their own countries, they would have access to modernity, to development, to stability. I had to agree that those things were certainly lacking now. But this is the danger of the work we do. Indigenous people don't see the value of the work done by the locals; they only see the value in work done by outsiders. In South Sudan, when I had a very similar conversation with village leaders, I pointed out the work that the local health-care providers were doing and was told, "But it is of no value; after all, it is here." Still, I know that when I leave, I will have helped to create value locally, and eventually the people will come to realize that.

The Azande "orphans" have not had the advantage of the great press that made the Lost Boys of South Sudan so well known around the world. The guilt of the Western nations from standing by during the savage oppression of the Sudanese Bantu people encouraged a push for adopting the Lost Boys, and many have been brought to the United States for resettlement and education. But the Azande haven't enjoyed the same PR campaign, despite suffering similar oppression for decades. There have been no Sundance Film Festival documentaries like *God Grew Tired of Us*, and no bestselling books like *What Is the What* or *They Poured Fire on Us from the Sky*. No amnesty has been granted to the thousands of Zande refugees in the CAR, as it was to the Dinka or Nuer. Because of Joseph Kony and the LRA, the plight of the Azande and others who live at the pole of inaccessibility may be slightly better known, but the support they have received is nowhere near the level granted to the Sudanese Lost Boys. Any group that has captured the interest and imagination of the West in the "branding" that comes from the media of their "poster child" status is unlikely to give up that advantage by pointing out that there are many other destitute peoples that share the fate of poverty and despair in the pole of inaccessibility. Each of these "orphan" groups seeks the "special" status that might lead to its "adoption" by first-world advocates. Each ethnic clan-sized group tries to emphasize its uniqueness through its own compelling story, as a very charismatic "numerator" drawn out from the anonymous mass of the "denominator" of the world's mind-numbing numbers of the global poor and disadvantaged. "We alone deserve to get everything you have got" was the translation of a phrase once uttered as a claim upon my beneficence in South Sudan. It certainly does not hurt to try, since some of us may be so naïve or guilty as to take up that demand, often uttered in Biblical language about "brothers' keepers." Few of these special potential adoptees are eager to call attention to other similarly disadvantaged brethren, making them "accessible" to the limited aid that might dilute the advantage that comes with the tenuous attention attracted to their own plight.

At this point, Joe proceeded to stand up and, with innocent naïveté, said essentially, "I had never heard of you before. But I'm a filmmaker, and now that I'm here, the whole world is going to know about you and supply you with the same aid that these excellent people have provided." I wanted to pull him down into his seat. He had announced that he was the media that would create their brand and that the world would be coming to their aid.

Over the course of the evening, the locals expressed surprise at the qualifications some of us carried. They were hoping to attain a few of these some day, even though some were aware that ours is a highly regulated and restricted environment that is virtually out of reach for anyone here. Long gone are the days when the hardworking houseboy might be taken into the Bible school here and then at some future point might be sponsored to visit the United States and possibly attend some similar school there. When they see that I have achieved a few extra degrees, many are eager—as were the much more aggressive Dinka when I visited them—to become my dependents so that I might carry them through all the advanced courses as their sponsor—"like a Dinka Uncle," one of them said to me.

Our final operating day began somewhat slowly. First, our team finally received messages on their phones this morning; the reception on the phone cards they had purchased in Entebbe finally went through, at the very end of our trip. They could talk with their home bases, even if it meant waking up spouses at 1:00 a.m. We also unpacked and assembled the operating microscope and its power source and began with the three cataract patients we had selected. This meant we could only use one table instead of the two-table rodeo we had been running. We began with other operations at noon and worked after the cataractectomies to make up for lost time.

A woman I had seen in the clinic the day before had a large, fixed, and firm breast cancer, but had no nodes or other evidence that it had spread. So we did a quadrantectomy, or a partial mastectomy, to remove the tumor intact, but not much more than that. The tamoxifen, a breast cancer drug, was still there from my last visit to Zemio. Later, if there were any evidence of spread, Ambroise could get it to her on the next connection between Zemio and Obo.

A woman came to us complaining of small insects invading her ear. She was convincing, especially when she pulled out a small scrap of paper with what looked like miniature bees inside. I suggested we drown them and drain them out of her ear with mineral oil, since I doubted they could swim. Claudia had a similar insect observation; she had seen a swarm of bees in the latrine. She asked if someone who used the latrine might have diabetes, a reasonable question since bees are attracted to the excess glucose in the urine of people with diabetes. Years ago, that was the test for the condition. However, no one with juvenile diabetes in this region would have survived long enough to come see us, and no one here has a lifestyle of surfeit that would cause them to develop type II diabetes. So the bees must just be following us Westerners into the outhouse!

It took a while to get to the large number of patients we had. Having heard they could get free surgical care, they were still arriving from far and wide. With the AIM AIR pilot arriving here early in the morning after an overnight in Zemio, according to a message relayed by Mary Anne Harris, the pressure was on to finish out our last day strong.

"We will never see the 'last patient,'" I told the team members, "so don't try to convince yourself that we will complete the work here or anywhere. As long as you are still standing here, having done more in less time than you could have dreamed possible, there will still be patients on their way to get here, and a sighting of you is all they need to expect the care they seek. I have had patients come to me at the airplane, expecting to be treated as we are loading up for the flight out. For them, the clinic is open as long as you are visible anywhere near it."

This time we had to worry less about the latecomers, since the ground team with the Zemio medical clinic vehicle and all of the supplies will still be here. When we go wheels-up in the morning—presuming we do—the team of Ambroise, Isaiah, Celestine, Sacco, as well as the others of the Obo staff, such as John the Dentiste, will still be here to fix the stragglers. They may also be joined by the US Army Special Forces medics, who might return to assist Ambroise and company for the few days more that they will remain in Obo. The Zemio team will then pack up the rest of the stock. With the vehicle, escort, and fuel paid for, they will work their way through Mboki, Jemma, and Mboosa before returning to Zemio.

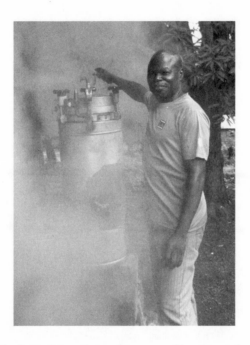

John the Dentiste vents steam from our wood-burning autoclave.

I will await their lead before coming up with plans for the next trip, which will surely involve a return mobile surgical mission; however, I hope at that time that there will be *zareda* (Pazande for "peace") enough to allow a hunt and leisure enough to explore a bit of this exotic and remote pole of inaccessibility.

As we tried to sleep on our last night in Obo, we were serenaded by an all-night tropical downpour. We listened to the chirping chorus of termite-stuffed frogs and toads. But even that chorus was eventually drowned out by the thunder and heavy drumming of rain on the roof.

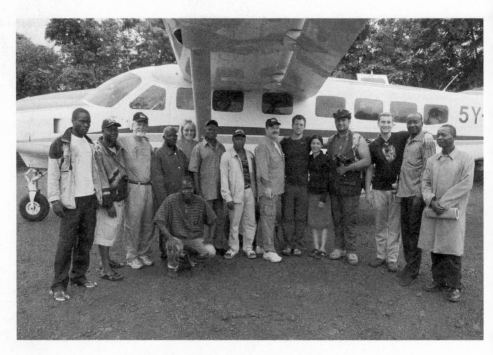

The whole team poses for a picture just before takeoff.

CHAPTER TWELVE

OBO TO ADDIS ABABA

June 16–17, 2012, Obo, CAR, to Entebbe, Uganda,
to Addis Ababa, Ethiopia

WE WERE ONCE AGAIN IN ENTEBBE, UGANDA, ON THE GREAT LAKE Victoria, having left Obo early in the morning and traveled by way of Zemio, Assa, Arua, and Banda. We covered a lot of geography, but not so much as we would cover the next day, as we traversed three continents in our travels home. What we saw was a whole lot of Zande land in the Central African Republic and the Democratic Republic of the Congo, while revisiting decades-old memories. For the refugeed Azande, these lands held memories of better times, when attention from the outside world came from benign and helpful groups, not from brutal raiders.

We had breakfast and then gathered at the runway, where we were swarmed by the team at Obo and the Zemio group before they went to do consultations, hernia repairs, and other operations over the coming days. The US Army Special Forces arrived in a truck, toting Mark Pearson along as well.

I said we would soon hear the turbine of the incoming plane, and moments later, at about 6:35 a.m., the white Cessna 208 Caravan came in low, made a short flyby of the runway to check out the mud puddles, and then touched down. When we got to the edge of the runway, we saw that it was not Jon Hildebrandt in the pilot's seat but Jim Streit, a great guy from Chicago who has been out in the field as long as many of the missionary kids. We loaded our 160 kilograms of freight, a load that had been much reduced after we donated all of our medical and surgical equipment. This was the first time that Jim Streit had met Mark Pearson, despite frequent radio contact and stories told back and forth by mutual friends. This is a fairly common occurrence here; consider that I had never met the Harrises, despite the fact that we had been working in nearby villages for over twenty years. They were actually closer to the pole of inaccessibility.

Jim carried parcels from Mary Anne Harris to people in Obo, including letters and supplies for the Bible school.

We all took photos and swapped email and postal addresses. There were lots of promises about future missions and the timing of the next grand safari. Each of the team members talked about how *stunned* they were by the rate, the volume, the intensity, and the success of this surgical mission, and our hopes for still further progress. We piled aboard the plane, bounced around the mud puddles, and waved as we took off from Obo for the thirty-minute trip to Zemio, our port of emigration.

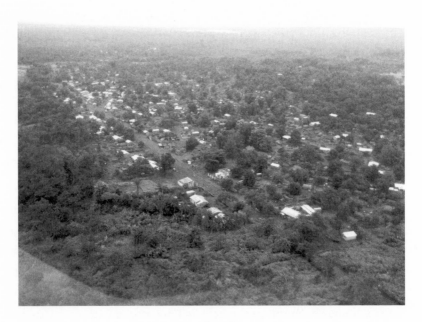

Zemio, from above.

We were on approach to Zemio, coming down the slope, when I yelled, "The goats!" A herd of goats had wandered onto the airfield, gathering right at the touchdown point and not getting out of the way, even with the noise of the approaching plane. Jim pulled the nose up, leveled off, made a circle over the town, and then made a pass at the runway from the opposite end to touch down and roll into a now-goat-free zone. African ecology, one. The finest of Cessna technology, zero.

Dan ran the passports to the "emigration officer" in the shack near the runway, while Jim loaded our fuel tanks and I rummaged in the hangar for the bag we had left behind. As I pulled out the bag, I found a bundle wrapped in newspaper stuck on top. I unwrapped it and found a handcrafted knife with a smooth handle and tailored blade. There was no signature, but it was hardly necessary. It was Merci Andre's handiwork. The knife now rests in a place of honor in the Derwood game room, where I am reminded of Merci Andre each time I pass it.

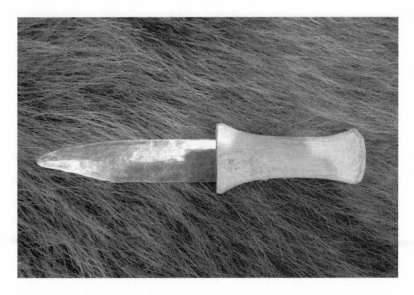

The knife made for me by Merci Andre, at home on a bearskin rug in the Derwood game room.

I pulled out my first set of running shoes, in which I had arrived, and took off the ones I had been wearing for two weeks. They'd taken me through two ORs and many mud puddles.

Jim had passed on a request that I meet with Jean Marco at the Zemio airfield. Jean Marco came on the run with a plastic bag wrapped around mail to be forwarded to his two daughters, who were in school in Isiro, DRC, and to his son, who has graduated but is now seeking a postgraduate sponsor. He also had letters he asked me to send to friends in the United States. I remembered to ask him about Kongonyesi, another Zande from Assa with whom I had shared many hunts. When we were in Zemio in January, he had greeted us at the airfield. He became my private patient when I learned that he had bilateral hernias. Jean Marco smiled when I asked about Kongonyesi and said, "Back to Assa!" My Assa friends were making their own decisions about returning home, despite the fact that they did not yet have clearance from the UNHCR, which has declared the area unsafe for repatriation. I told Jean Marco in broken French that we were about to do a flyover of Assa, and that we would try to discover who and what was left there now. Perhaps our next visit might take place there. I handed him a copy of *Out of Assa: Heart of the Congo* and said something as close as I could get in Pazande about going "into Assa—like next year, in Jerusalem!"

To be sure we had cleared all the items and expenses for the Zemio mission station, I asked if we could call Les and Mary Anne Harris on the plane's radio; they had a radio in the house. We totaled up Zemio room and board for seven people over seven nights, and I was reminded that I needed to pay the amount in cash. I asked if I could send US currency to Les and Mary Anne by way of Jean Marco; they could then give the cash to Zapai. But Jim floated me the cash, very graciously, and I planned on giving Jim a check made out to AIM for the flights and balances. I still didn't know the amount for room and board at Obo, which would be added to my account later. Much of the overage would float on my AIM account until I received the bills at Derwood.

Les and Mary Anne told us that after we left (and Bruce, our snake-phobe, should be grateful for the timing) they killed a black mamba that had crawled into the kitchen where we had been spending time just about a week before. It got Bruce thinking better of Obo over Zemio, despite the nighttime appearance of snakes on the hunt for toads.

After saying our final good-byes, our plane took off, and I asked Jim if we might buzz around Assa, only about sixty miles southeast of Zemio, just to see it again and to let them know we are thinking of them and that we will someday return, possibly on the next trip. It wasn't much outside of our flight plan toward Arua, and he agreed to take the detour. We lined up for Assa and headed down over the *mungas*—footprint-like expanses of hardened lava that once flowed from vast shield volcanoes of the central African "Mountains of the Moon." We came in low, banked around, and saw people outside the school and the church and "hospital," as well as over near the main mission house. We turned around and buzzed low over the airstrip and right over Zara, a marshy water hole where runoff from the mungas collects. This may be the source of the mysterious Assa River, which flows underground, in the domed cavities beneath the mungas, before joining the Uele River. Jim held us at a thousand feet as we made a long sightseeing cruise. I kept my head pressed to the Plexiglas, looking for the animal life I had known at these sites.

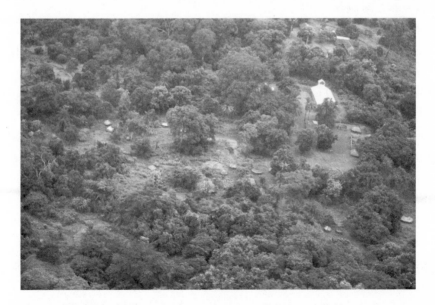

Assa station, appearing much as it did when I was last there, possibly the last European visitor. It is still largely evacuated, but there were people in the compound who waved at us as we circled above.

I hoped to see something big enough to share with the team, like elephants, but I didn't have luck there. I did spot Cape buffalo (*nyati*), with their large, curling horns, in singles and pairs. The thick green cover was so lush and dense that only at water holes could we spot anything. I saw several defassa waterbuck, which are large and have horns that curve slightly out and back and point toward the sky, and a few *bodi*, or bushbuck, and a giant forest hog, a zigba. Bruce confirmed most of the sightings; however, the others did not see the animals, and Joe had gone toward the back of the plane to get a good photograph of the flight over Assa.

As we climbed toward 13,500 feet, Jim learned that I had spent a lot of time in the right seat, having once been a certified pilot, and had also been an aviation medical examiner. He asked if I wanted to take control of the Cessna. I said it would be a pleasure, particularly so that I could report back to my eldest grandson, Andrew, that I had once again flown in the airspace where I had done most of my early flying. Andrew William Geelhoed had a pilot's license before he could drive, and I knew he would have loved this experience. The yoke was getting hard to hold on course and at altitude, so I spun the trim tabs a bit to even us out.

We landed briefly in Arua to refuel and check on a few things and then were up in the air again on our way to Entebbe. I did much more flying on the longer flight out of Arua, crossing the White Nile and the big Lake Kyoga. We had to bob and weave around tropical thunderheads, and skirting some of the big cloud banks made for a bumpy ride. My drowsy passengers did not seem to notice—or at least they didn't say anything. I told Joe that uncertified surgical operators have been doing a good job taking care of patients, so the passengers could feel comfortable that a no-longer-certified pilot could get them safely to Entebbe.

We flew directly over the mission station at Banda, which is on a hill that rises up partially from the surrounding DRC bush. It was at Banda, with its extensive schools and a hospital, where I had once operated with the scrub nurse who put her hand on a green mamba slithering over the sterile Mayo stand. A more bittersweet memory was that I had operated with Andre the Dentiste there. His father had melanoma of the foot (in one of the very few places that an African is likely to develop a melanoma, a "melanotic whitlow"—under the great toe nailbed, which lacks protective pigment) that had metastasized to the groin and lungs. I had one single chemotherapeutic agent, cyclophosphamide—an agent not very effective against melanoma but wonderfully effective against Burkitt's lymphoma, the most common form of cancer among children in this part of Africa. I had just discovered a young girl with the disease in the clinic. She was blessed by the presence of Andre's father, who generously gave up the single treatment we had and offered it to her instead. However, the girl's mother could make no decisions as to whether her daughter could receive this highly effective treatment until the Zande elders of Banda consulted a diviner to determine who it was that caused this illness to fall upon her and whether she should receive the medicine. While her mother waited anxiously for the elders to schedule the divination, the girl died.

I was still thinking of this while leaving the Banda hilltop compound behind. Flying along with my hands on the controls of a simple and efficient device, I considered how we had been operating. Our techniques were hardly rocket science; they were very human applications of knowledge to human problems—goiters or prostatism or getting from point A to point B across the jungle. We do what we can and let the Creator move us toward ends that are not our own.

With the great Lake Victoria in our view, we began our descent. The TAWS voice squawked that we were below five hundred feet above ground; she is as hard to argue with as the Australian woman's voice in the GPS of my Audi A4 back home. We landed next to the big Soviet-era Ilyushin aircraft, painted in UN white, and saw the Ethiopian Airlines plane we would take the next day waiting for us on the tarmac. We paid another $50 to immigrate into Uganda for just one night, and met our driver, Jemima, who was holding up a sign that said, "Dr. Glen and Team Central Inn."

At the hotel, Deo, our "arranger," came by and put the four guys in apartments, the Arch Apartments, behind Central Inn. Claudia and Leenta checked into one room at the inn, and I into another. I typed up my letter recounting the trip for all our friends and supporters at home. We had a good dinner at the inn and then turned in early to get some much-needed rest before another long day of traveling.

I spent most of my twenty-four hours in Entebbe struggling to do two simple things: pay bills without currency and send one email.

When we first checked into the Central Inn, the front desk clerk announced that the credit card machine was not working. "I'll come down in an hour and we will try again," I said. Of course, I wasn't surprised to hear the news, given what had happened on our last trip through, but I thought that I would try anyway.

"It has not been working for two weeks," the clerk told me.

"Okay, I will give you a check."

"Let me see the check . . . Okay . . . No, not okay. Do you have a traveler's check?"

"No." *Who uses traveler's checks any more?*

"You will have to pay in Ugandan shillings or US dollars."

I essentially replied, "You are unlucky, since the CAR folk, who also do not accept checks or plastic, got to me first and relieved me of all US dollars."

"You will then go to a bank and bring me cash."

"I don't believe there is a bank open on Saturday evening," I said.

"Okay, then you can do it tomorrow morning."

"Isn't it less likely that they would be open on Sunday morning?"

"Deo will arrange it for you."

So, we may have moved to upmarket Uganda, the Pearl of Africa, but that does not mean that transactions are any less complicated. This is still Africa, and explanations of problems are offered in deliberate, and often tortured, English. The clerk and I had our conversation in front of signs advertising the fact that the inn honors MasterCard, American Express, and Visa, yet the clerk seemed to have no clue how to do so. So, I am a debtor.

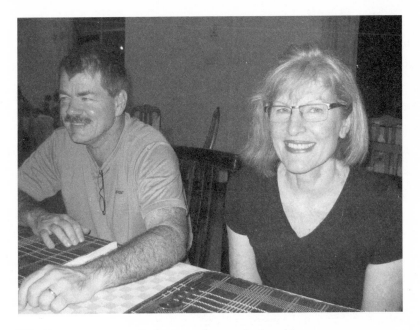

Bruce and Leenta at dinner at the Central Inn.

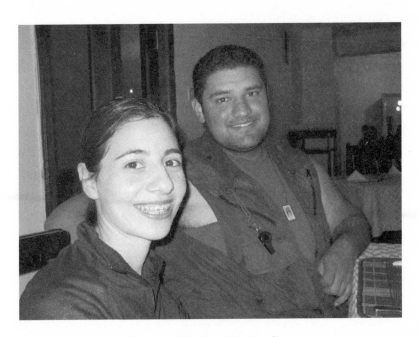

Claudia and Joe, also at the Central Inn.

The ridiculousness continued after dinner. We waited for a bill, but none came, so I went upstairs to my room. About ten minutes later a woman knocked on the door and handed me a bill for thousands of shillings, or about US $69. I said she should add it to the room charge and it would be settled together with the hotel charge. Okay. But a few minutes later, there was another knock at the door. The same woman told me she needed to be paid with cash right now. I explained that she was far too late. My $100 bill from the Harrises was still in my pocket, but it was my emergency get-out-of-Africa stock.

I was working on an email summary of our experience at about ten o'clock when the phone rang. It was the front desk. Why had I not taken a taxi to the bank and withdrawn cash to pay my bills? the woman asked. I explained that I rather doubted there would be many banks open at ten o'clock on Saturday night, and that since they were holding my credit cards as security, I would see what I could do in the morning. Okay.

The next morning, I met Leenta and Claudia at a good breakfast buffet, which I had forgotten was part of our hotel payment. I went to the front desk and learned, as I suspected, that there were no banks open and, of course, no machines that are advertised as ATMs work any better than the nonfunctioning credit card readers at the front desk. So I had no choice but to scrounge enough money for the hotel payment from the team members. Thankfully, Leenta was generous with her own $100 emergency bill. I pulled out the Harrises' $100 bill and gave it and Leenta's money to the clerks at the front desk. I had expected this to represent a triumph of solvency. Instead the clerks stood around examining the two bills. They rejected one, since it was not printed after 2010—their cutoff for acceptance. The second bill was printed after 2010—but it had a corner folded over and turned down and thus was unacceptable. "Okay, guys," I said, "you are simply out of luck." But Leenta and Claudia came to the rescue, giving up the last of their cash to cover the bill. I planned to reimburse each when we returned to the States.

We had planned to take a quick tour of Entebbe, or of Lake Victoria, or wherever Deo could take us, before heading out to the airport for our flight and three continents' worth of travel. We were heading to the van when Deo, who knew that I'd had no currency the night before, came to me and asked for $200 for the four rooms at the Arch Apartments. If I did not have money for the Central Inn, how would I have generated any for the Arch Apartments overnight? After telling the team of our impasse, I offered him the Harrises' $100 bill (the one printed after 2010) with the corner smoothed out, and it was combined with a number of tens and fives from the team.

Once we'd cleared the bill, we piled into the van for the tour.

We drove around the cement ramp down to Lake Victoria, where there is a ferry that carries vehicles across to Tanzania. We watched a boatload of lumber being off-loaded; the workers simply threw all the boards into the lake, picked them up as they floated to shore, and then loaded them on a truck. A long dugout was taking on passengers, who were crouched side by side in the middle of the boat—there was a motorbike up on the stern of the dugout and two goats at the bow, bleating out into Lake Victoria under overcast skies.

We drove around a lot of gated communities that were full of, primarily, UN employees. These individuals lived high on the hill overlooking Lake Victoria, above the small markets and the shantytown below. It seemed there were more people living *off* poverty than *in* it here. We passed the offices of a long list of NGOs, including the Jane Goodall Institute, the Uganda Viral Research Institute, the Medical Research Council of England, an AIDS hospital and AIDS orphans' home, and many other volunteer groups with names that sounded like they hoped to restore the world to perfection, even amid the squalor of muddy roads and corrugated pan roofing.

The Pearl of Africa is a good place, but it is also overrun with NGOs, relief agencies, and church organizations, and for one big reason: There is no need of translation. English is commonly spoken here. Because of the language divide, the CAR, the DRC, and Chad get only a fraction of the interest that Uganda, Kenya, and Tanzania do, particularly from missionaries. I saw busloads of church groups driving through Entebbe, as many are coming out for their summer missions programs.

The development is vastly different here than in other parts of Africa, and not one of our group would have been aware of that had they not been to the CAR. At least we were not on tour in Africa for self-gratification alone.

I made the decision that we would bypass the botanical gardens and go to the Uganda Wildlife Education Centre—essentially a zoo—which was laid out on the shores of Lake Victoria. As we entered, we saw signs asking for memberships to preserve the wildlife, like the rhinos. There are no rhinos of either black or white varieties in the whole nation of Uganda, except in zoos. We also saw a sign proclaiming that the center accepted American Express and MasterCard and Visa—at last. As foreign nationals, it cost $15 for each of us, a total of $105, so I gave them my AmEx and Visa and MasterCard and all of them were run through the machine, "which has not been working." Led by Dan Vryhof, the team came up with the cash to get us into the zoo. But their funds were now about as tapped out as my own.

Deo asked whether we would be having lunch at the restaurant overlooking Lake Victoria, and then he added that I needed to give him $40 for the van and fuel for our excursion. Although I might have expected this, it did not occur to him that I still had no currency. When it came time to part, I gave Deo the last cash I had, a $10 bill. Deo looked at it and said it was of no use to him since it was engraved before 2010, so I took it back—after all, it was worth $10 more to me than it was to him!

We saw penned-in giraffes and Livingstone's elands, Cape buffalo, warthogs, and a number of almost free-ranging birds, such as African crowned cranes, the emblematic totem of Uganda. As I watched them trying to jump the brush fence with clipped wings, I saw a flash of green above my head, and a gorgeous malachite kingfisher glided up into the tree. It is the leading candidate for my vote for the most spectacular bird that flies.

Soon we came upon another of the most spectacular birds of Uganda— the shoebill stork. We had gone a long way out of our way to spot one in

Zambia on a brief birding safari once and had never found one. One of the indigenous guides on the trip had smiled and said, "Ah, yes, very delicious!"

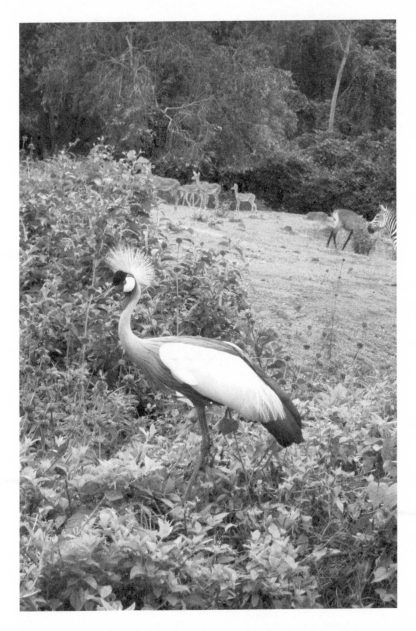

The African crowned crane (Balearica pavonina), Uganda's totemic emblem.

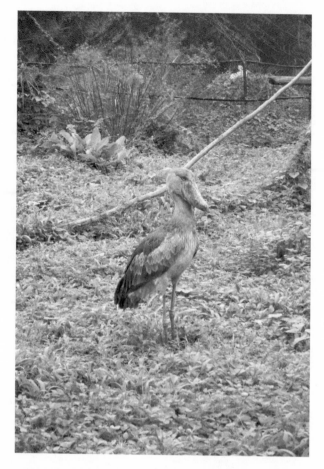

The shoebill stork (Balaeniceps rex), another emblematic bird of Uganda.

We saw a male and female lion, spotted hyenas, a large colony of chimpanzees on an island, spotted-necked otters cavorting and standing up like meerkats to stare at us before diving into the water in their swirling corkscrew dives, and big Nile crocodiles with mouths gaping open to thermoregulate. We admired reedbuck, impala, Burchell's zebras, the rock python and Gabon viper, and a dozen more birds.

Joe was lugging around all of his equipment—despite not taking any photos—and that meant he was always lagging (and was also the one who got frisked in security more than anyone else). He was worried about his limited capacity, since he had wanted to use my laptop before we boarded to download his interviews again. I had to say no. No way could I let him bleed the energy out of my laptop before being sequestered for sixteen hours on an airplane with whatever battery juice remained from the last charge. So he took most of the morning to set up, and then interviewed Claudia in front of Lake Victoria. I thought a better backdrop would be the Elder Tree—a ficus well over a hundred years old and a huge climax forest specimen, under which elders would gather to dispense justice and wisdom to the young. I was supposed to be interviewed before we left, but Joe seemed always short of equipment and time. However, he interviewed Leenta later at the Central Inn.

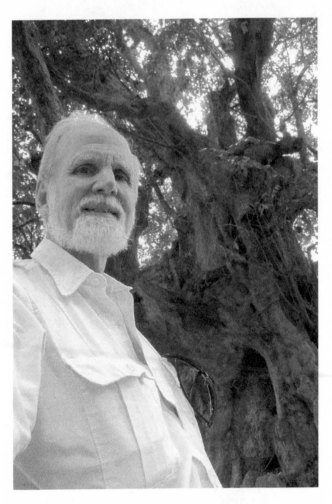

The magnificent centenarian—the Elder Tree.

We sat on the porch of the restaurant at lunch and admired the view of vast Lake Victoria. The weather was almost pleasant, thanks to the lake breezes. We watched kingfishers, egrets, hammerkopfs, and lots of noisy Egyptian geese flying in to freeload off the park's food supply. We watched two men in a dugout canoe, one paddling and the other casting a net in a perfect arc over the shoals of Lake Victoria, a timeless silhouette from the valley where man was born.

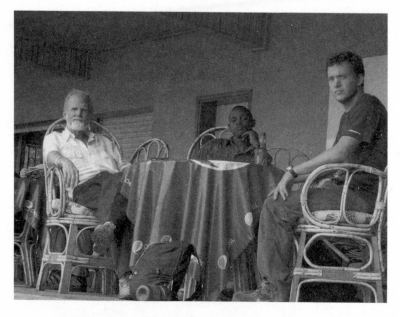

I, Deo, and Dan enjoy a little R&R on the Lake Victoria lakeshore,
at the Uganda Wildlife Education Centre.

As we headed back to the hotel, I said that I hoped to send my single email message. I had tried the night before, to no avail. In both the Central Inn and the Arch Apartments, we saw signs offering Internet access. After a score of attempts two weeks before, I had been able to send out only a brief message that we had arrived in Entebbe—a miracle of communication that would've been simply accepted as an everyday occurrence elsewhere in the world. But it was an elusive goal this time.

When we got back to the hotel, Josh VanderWall and I went to the Arch Apartments, from which he had sent a series of successful emails. Josh connected new wires and worked on the modem and used his special skills to achieve absolutely no connection. He stayed with it longer than I would have, and we learned again the African lesson of maintaining an infinite threshold for frustration. We came back over to the Central Inn and Claudia found six different servers there, but none were accessible. Last night she had found one named Lynx, accessible only on the upper floors, so up we went. I tried to log in to my GWU account—and got it! I pushed "send" and off the email went. A single message had gone out twice, from even this "developed" part of central Africa, coming and going, taking only a day each in their sending.

So, after a full day trying to pay bills without currency, and the rest of the same day trying to send one simple email, what the team has learned is that in Africa, there is often a failure to communicate.

With two successes that had taken all day—but that would've taken two minutes in the well-wired world—we were able to pack the van and leave with Deo for the airport. We got checked in at the last minute and flew the two hours together to Addis Ababa. When we arrived, we went to the transit lounge for the compulsory purchase of Ethiopian coffee.

When it came time to board the Ethiopian Airlines flight back to the United States, I got the last bit of excitement the trip would offer. At the gate check-in desk, an attendant told me that my luggage had been pulled, and I had to go to the secured luggage area to claim it for inspection. I had never wandered around in the bowels of Bole International Airport before, and apparently neither had the security agent who was accompanying me. After walking through the underbelly of the passenger waiting lounges, watching big trolleys and conveyor belts feed luggage through X-ray machines and into bins to be loaded, we found a higher office overlooking the floor and its conveyor belts. A woman motioned me to get my Safari Club International bag from the belt, and then they took everything out of it, emptying Dopp kits and camera bags from the blue duffel. When she took the backpack out, I knew what she was after. She removed the clothes and triumphantly pulled out one zigba tusk.

"What is this and where did you get it?"

I told her I had come from a humanitarian mission in the CAR and that this warthog tusk was a gift from the people there. The security agent said, "It did not originate in Ethiopia, so it is of no consequence. They must have thought it was contraband ivory being smuggled."

I looked at him and said, "They must have rather small elephants in the CAR!" They all laughed and thanked me for my patience. They put it back in the bag, and I was led back up the stairs and into the security line to be scanned once again.

So, I was the last passenger on this Ethiopian Airlines flight. It was a fitting conclusion to the mission—the collision of modernity and high technology with the product of the hunter-gatherer instincts that governed much of our interactions.

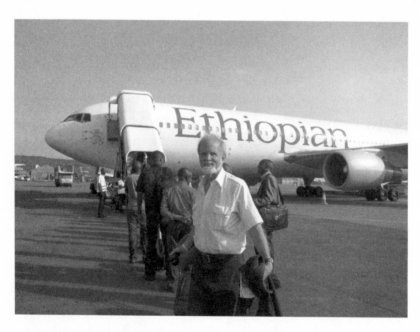

Takeoff at Entebbe. Departing Africa yet again—but I always come back.

EPILOGUE

In 2007, I was leading a medical mission in the Kauda Valley of the Nuba Mountains in Sudan. The people in the region, the Nuba tribe, became the victims of state-sponsored genocidal attacks beginning in the early 1990s, when General Omar Bashir took control of the country and fanned the flames of ethnic tension between nomadic Arabic-speaking tribes and African Bantu pastoralists. Since then, there have been brief intervals of lesser violence of the Sudanese war, but the Nuba people still face regular attacks by the government.

We were there during a lull in the violence, a few years after Bashir began allowing relief workers into the region. We were working in the German Emergency Doctors Hospital, a clinic near Kauda. When we heard that the few low buildings housed a fairly well-equipped operating room, we were excited to begin using it as soon as possible. Unfortunately, that would never happen.

The chief, although temporary, nurse did not want us to see the basic OR, and she certainly did not want us to utilize it.

"Why?" I asked, dumbfounded.

"There is nothing we can do for these people," she said. "I don't want to be stuck here with post-op care of surgical patients. And I don't want these people to expect a surgical cure when we will not be able to do any such thing. But they will return and remind us that simple operations can be done, since they had been done."

Not only were we not allowed to use the operating room or to teach indigenous health-care workers, we were not allowed to treat certain conditions either. A man from the Nuba tribe came in with all the classic symptoms of tuberculosis—a common event. Global research shows that TB "is second only to HIV/AIDS as the greatest killer worldwide due to a single infectious agent," according to the World Health Organization (WHO). And it's estimated that 1.4 million people died from TB in 2011. Sub-Saharan Africa had the greatest proportion of new cases per capita. But here's the fascinating item: TB is recognizable, preventable, and curable, which is part of the reason that the mortality rate has dropped by 41 percent since 1990 (WHO, "Global Tuberculosis Report 2012"). So when I saw this man, I discussed beginning treatment right away with the nurse.

Her response astounded me, although maybe I should not have been surprised. She told me that the hospital wouldn't treat the man. "Why not?" I asked.

"Treating him will take nine months, and he may die anyway. We would have to support him and his family. They're going to come to depend on us. There's really nothing we can do to help these people."

She repeated this sentiment multiple times in the days we were there. The phrase will stay with me forever, conveying a sentiment that I have spent my professional life railing against, even if I didn't realize it until that moment.

I pushed forward. I wrote up the patient's diagnosis and prescribed his treatment. The nurse withheld the treatment. The patient lingered for a few days and then died as we were leaving.

A health-care worker refuses to treat a curable illness. Local governments refuse to provide basic services, turning against their citizens rather than supporting them. Foreign governments refuse to come to the aid of certain oppressed peoples. While there are larger sociopolitical issues at play that are difficult to resolve, why do they refuse to attempt to solve fairly basic health-care problems, particularly when the problems are sitting right in front of them? Because the need is enormous and seemingly insatiable, and once help is available, people may abandon their fatalism and rush forward with more problems to unburden on health-care providers. Nobody wants to become entangled, but they do little to prevent that entanglement; when they do offer aid, they rarely do so in a way that encourages independence. "There's really nothing we can do to help these people" has become a self-fulfilling prophecy.

However, that tide has been shifting, and more and more organizations are discovering better paths, recognizing the importance of education and cooperation, understanding the cultural differences that require a different approach.

The German Emergency Doctors mission was to eventually turn the clinics they had established in Africa over to indigenous health-care workers. Apparently, the clinic we were in was a "problem child." Still, most can see the wisdom of teaching a man to fish, with whatever pole and bait are immediately available.

I've seen the pitfalls. I've heard the pleas for more help. It's the biggest danger of the work we do on our missions. We try so hard to keep the focus on enhancing the skills of the local health-care workers, yet both the people we treat and the overburdened health-care providers often see us as their saviors, and they believe that our presence means that a flood of greater first-world aid is coming. That is a pipe dream. Despite the fact that we must constantly battle those perceptions, I believe that "these people" can be helped and can become independent, using aid when they desperately need it but not relying on it. And through my belief, I hope that they will come to believe in themselves and their capability to overcome the hurdles they face on their own.

The planning for our next trip to the CAR began on the road between Zemio and Obo. But it hit a snag when, in March 2013, a new faction, the Séléka coalition, took control of the government, ousting François Bozizé, who had been president for ten years—an ineffectual ten years. For months, I tried to communicate with Ambroise via email. Before the overthrow, the Séléka militia was working its way through the eastern part of the country, and we were unsure whether they had taken Zemio or whether our friends were safe. Eventually, the rebels had turned toward Bangui and then the coup was over fairly quickly. A few weeks later, I finally heard from Ambroise. He was safe, the villages were stable, and life was continuing on—because what happens in Bangui really has little effect on the lives of the people in the eastern CAR.

Whether they realize it or not, they are already independent, at least from their own government. Who knows whether that will change with the new government, or how long the new government will be in power.

But Mission to Heal must keep moving forward, because we also are independent. We have been working on a grand plan—the development of mobile surgical units that can be transported across countries and continents, docking at local clinics in villages across the world. They will become spectacular training centers, allowing us to work with more indigenous caregivers in more towns because we will have to rely less on expensive or uncertain transportation of people and supplies. And it will allow us to spend more time in each area because we will have more supplies with us, not simply whatever we can pack into some duffel bags.

More important, with the development of mobile surgical units, we can recruit more first-world physicians who are intrigued by what I do but are wary of jumping in without access to more modern facilities and supplies— such as electricity. I recognize that not everybody is as comfortable operating under a tree as I have, out of necessity, become. A regular rotation of volunteer physicians and students in larger numbers can keep the programs sustainable and can help train local providers in different types of surgical procedures. And this seventy-year-old volunteer will not be able to withstand the strenuous effort of these missions indefinitely.

Patients, too, would be transformed by the regular appearance of mobile units. For indigenous patients to gain access to care that could be life-saving or life-improving, they must be aware of it and it must be local. Training providers in more than just two villages in a region, or even an entire country, makes care more accessible to all. It removes the necessity to travel unrealistic distances, to dislocate family members who must come along as caregivers, and to separate people from their basic livelihoods, without which they cannot survive.

As I write this, I'm preparing to transport all of the "software"—sutures, sponges, gowns, gloves—to the warehouse of the Medical Mission Hall of Fame Foundation in Toledo, Ohio. There, we'll meet a truck coming from Project SAVE in Chico, California, carrying operating tables, lights, and gurneys, as well as our new, big, diesel rescue truck being delivered from Iowa. The next step will be to procure the trailer that will become our two-table operating room and will be pulled behind the truck, its power source. The challenge has been to find vehicles that can handle the rough terrain of the places we go. Most vehicles can travel on the rough roads during the dry season in the equatorial zone, but during the rainy season, road traffic grinds to a halt. Disease processes do not. So the mobile units will be transferred to barges on the Amazon, the Nile, the Volta, and other major rivers and the oceans between islands. These floating facilities will continue operating through the rainy season.

In Toledo, we'll put a wrap on the truck with the logos of Mission to Heal and whatever other organizations want to be involved and then park it outside the offices of the Students for Medical Missions Symposium at the University of Toledo.

Participants from both missions to the CAR, as well as from others to South Sudan, Nigeria, Ghana, Ecuador, and the Philippines, will be attending. In late summer of 2013, we'll begin another annual journey around the world, first driving down to Sonora, Mexico, and then down to Ecuador, where we'll be working in the Amazon with the indigenous Shuar people and in the Andes with the Indian population. From there, we'll ferry the unit out to the Galápagos Islands to work with the twenty thousand people who live there, who are generally ignored. Then, the truck and trailer will be shipped across the Pacific to the Philippines, where we'll make a circuit of many of the islands, further developing the clinics that we set up in January 2010, 2011, 2012, and 2013. (I left for the Philippines directly after dropping Flore off in Kenya.)

After the Philippines, the path is uncertain as to schedule but fixed in destinations. The hope is to go to Nepal and India in the Himalayas, where missions are already scheduled, as funding permits. If not, we'll ship it straight to Africa and begin a safari that will lead us from Ghana, Nigeria, and Chad to the CAR and through all of the towns Ambroise visited on his return trip to Zemio, setting up clinics along the way. We already have requests for mobile mission "dockings" in Nigeria, Ghana, Chad, South Sudan, Tanzania, Kenya,

Ethiopia, and of course, the CAR. A circuit in Asia is being developed for another mobile surgical unit.

In addition to questions of funding are questions of security. We cannot go to places that are so insecure that we risk being attacked. This was a problem on our most recent trip to South Sudan. I set up a clinic with supplies in one village and then traveled to another village to work there for a few days. When I returned to the first village on my way out, there was a man who needed an amputation after an accident that had crushed his leg months before, resulting in gangrene. I asked for the supplies to be prepared and was told we had none. How could that be, I asked—I'd just stocked them. Somebody had come through and pilfered them.

A few days later, security issues became more immediate. Just a couple of days after I put the seven members of my student team on the AIM AIR plane to begin their long trip homeward, I was caught in the crossfire of a burgeoning civil war. I lay in my tent with bullets from automatic weapons shredding the nylon above my head. I was pulled out of the area in a UN tank. As I tried to capture the unfolding events on film, the Sikh Indian soldiers in the tank were shouting at me to get down. The tank treads were clanking so loudly, I couldn't hear the fifty-caliber slugs hitting the steel plates around me. The UN Peacekeeping Force was being fired on. There does not seem to be any peace to be kept. It is likely that peace will first have to be made before the continuing carnage can be abated.

The final hurdle? A steady stream of volunteers. Calvin College is working toward developing the Mission to Heal Institute, through which students would receive college credit for their time spent on these missions. Other colleges are exploring similar programs. And with the support of organizations like NIFA, we'll continue to find other health-care professionals to assist us. The American College of Surgeons, through its Operation Giving Back, will supply qualified surgeons as teachers for indigenous workers.

We can "clone" the multiple experts at each level of service from the ongoing work of CinterAndes Foundation, with Dr. Edgar Rodas, the pioneer in the field of successful mobile surgical services in Ecuador with whom we have shared missions in all parts of Ecuador, now poised to join us in internationalizing our global mobile missions.

But our biggest sources of volunteers are returnees and the friends and family of past participants. Claudia continues to be a major volunteer for M2H and will join us on future missions. Dan Vryhof's brother Nick joined us on missions in 2013, and his father continues to be of great help through his service on our board and will join in the forthcoming missions in Ghana and the Himalayas. And Josh VanderWall's sister, who is a nurse, will be joining us on a trip to Africa. This trend is promising; it means we're doing something right.

I had hoped that Joe's promised documentary work would produce more word of mouth and encourage volunteers, but as of yet, we have seen not a single frame from him.

Delivering health care to the neediest people in the planet's "bottom billion" is not easy; as yet, it has not even developed into a cottage industry. But through ingenuity and improvisation and many workarounds to cover lacking skills and facilities, the local populations are devising systems to cope. These are the real heroes we should be helping. They must manage larger problems in greater numbers with far fewer resources. In this they are the experts, and we must learn from them.

So, we keep pushing forward, searching for the resources, the people, and the environments through which to continue our work.

Our trips to the CAR in 2012 were remarkable, mostly because of what was achieved with a small group of workers. We accomplished far more than we had dreamed possible. With the help of indigenous practitioners, the US Army Special Forces, the missionaries, AIM AIR, my talented team members, and the Azande people, we did much good and learned many lessons. It is likely that we will return to CAR, among others of the world's neglected peoples, but not as frequently or for as long as many would like, including me. There is always more to be done. We are all on a Mission to Heal, even at the pole of inaccessibility.

Gloria Dei!

Index

About the Author

DR. GLENN W. GEELHOED IS A REVERED HEALER. A RENOWNED surgeon, he was awarded his MD from University of Michigan and completed his surgical training at Harvard University. He is a specialist in infectious and tropical disease, having studied at the London School of Hygiene and Tropical Medicine. He has a passion for teaching and is an author, mountain climber, and marathon runner. For over forty years, he has led medical surgical missions to the most remote and often dangerous corners of the planet to treat the forgotten people of the world. His commitment to the poor and disenfranchised is legendary, and he is the recipient of numerous humanitarian awards, most notably those from the American College of Surgeons in 2009, the Medical Mission Hall of Fame Foundation in 2005, and the Kennedy Foundation in 2000. Multiple publications have been written about him, perhaps the most unique being the publications of Safari Club International, which recognized him for his "Blue Bag Missions" to Africa, on which he carried his medical supplies in the huge blue duffle bags donated by SCI and emblazoned with its logo.

George Washington University recently recognized Dr. Geelhoed for holding over thirteen educational degrees, yet he remains a student with an unquenchable thirst for understanding of this world, its people, and its values.

Mission To Heal, a medical surgical nonprofit organization dedicated to healing, teaching, and empowering, is his vision. Together with various teams organized under his direction, he has completed hundreds of medical missions and continues to do so to places like Ecuador, Nigeria, the CAR, India, and the Republic of South Sudan. A man of faith, he believes that all prayers are heard and that he himself has been saved to serve. Perhaps the best summation of his purpose is found in his own words: "I am an American who by some accident of birth has been the recipient of so many blessings that I have not even begun to repay the interest."

1/2014